THE NEW YOU

For both men and women, having "work done" on their foreheads, eyelids, cheeks, noses, lips, chins, breasts, tummies, thighs, and other body parts is becoming fairly commonplace. This accessible, easy-to-follow question-and-answer guide covers all the basics of cosmetic surgery and enables anyone to prepare for the experience with realistic expectations.

ARE YOU CONSIDERING COSMETIC SURGERY?

Gives answers to all your questions about:

- Liposuction
- Eyebrow-lifts
- Cheek and chin implants
- Double-chin removal
- Face sanding
- Laser and chemical peels
- Nose reshaping
- Ear setbacks
- Neck-lifts
- Breast surgeries
- Cosmetic dentistry
- Scar revisions
- Spider-vein removal

ARE YOU CONSIDERING
COSMETIC SURGERY?

ARTHUR W. PERRY, M.D., F.A.C.S.
AND ROBIN K. LEVINSON

AVON BOOKS ◆ NEW YORK

The ideas, procedures, and suggestions in this book are intended to supplement, not replace, the medical advice of a trained medical professional. All matters regarding your health require medical supervision. Consult your physician before adopting the suggestions in this book, as well as any condition that may require diagnosis or medical attention. The authors and publisher disclaim any liability arising directly or indirectly from the use of this book.

AVON BOOKS
A division of
The Hearst Corporation
1350 Avenue of the Americas
New York, New York 10019

Copyright © 1997 by Arthur W. Perry and Robin K. Levinson
Published by arrangement with the authors
Visit our website at http://www.AvonBooks.com
Library of Congress Catalog Card Number: 97-93172
ISBN: 0-380-79159-5

First Avon Books Printing: November 1997

AVON TRADEMARK REG. U.S. PAT. OFF. AND IN OTHER COUNTRIES, MARCA REGISTRADA, HECHO EN U.S.A.

Printed in the U.S.A.

WCD   10 9 8 7 6 5 4 3 2 1

I dedicate this book to my husband, Larry, for his support and devotion, and to my children, Zoe Mae and Aaron Joon, who continually remind me of my priorities.

—Robin K. Levinson

I dedicate this book to my wife, Bedonna, and to my parents, Dr. Michael and Harriet Perry, who have seen me through project after project and helped guide my career. I further dedicate this book to my children, Benjamin, Meredith, and Julia, for their love, patience, and understanding.

—Arthur W. Perry, M.D., F.A.C.S.

ACKNOWLEDGMENTS

We thank the following people who contributed to the research and writing of this book: Prosthodontist Stephen I. Hudis, D.D.S., for his invaluable contribution to the chapter on cosmetic dentistry; Michael M. Perry, D.D.S., for lending his time and expertise to the cosmetic dentistry chapter; Thomas J. Krizek, M.D., F.A.C.S., chief of plastic surgery at the University of South Florida; and Thomas J. Baker, M.D., F.A.C.S., and Howard Gordon, M.D., F.A.C.S., plastic surgeons affiliated with the University of Miami, for their teaching and influence; Pam Mayers, R.N., and rest of the office staff for going the extra mile; all the cosmetic surgery patients who shared their stories with candor and humor; and literary agent Judith Riven and Avon Books Editor Christine Zika for giving birth to this project.

CONTENTS

Contents

INTRODUCTION

An attorney has elective surgery to tighten her droopy eyelids. She is thirty-seven years old.

A fifty-year-old divorcee has fine lines around her mouth zapped by a laser and her own fat injected into her lips to create a fashionable "pouty" look.

Competing in the job market with people half his age, a fifty-two-year-old unemployed accountant has liposuction to eliminate his "love handles."

As cosmetic surgery becomes more refined, less traumatic, and more accessible, scenarios like these are becoming increasingly familiar. Ordinary people—no longer just the super-rich and famous—are flocking to aesthetic plastic surgeons in record numbers. Physicians, in turn, are offering an ever-widening array of age-defying, beauty-enhancing procedures.

Despite its growing popularity and acceptance among the mainstream, cosmetic surgery is still major surgery. Most patients are delighted with their results. But others have been disappointed or even horrified. By arming yourself with the information contained in this book, there is a greater chance that you will be counted among the happy, satisfied patients.

Depending on whose data you believe, anywhere from

500,000 to 2.6 million Americans went under the cosmetic knife in 1994 alone. At any given moment, several million people are trying to decide whether aesthetic surgery is right for them. Countless others have already decided they want it, but have no idea where to turn. This book will enlighten people in both categories. It answers all your questions about cosmetic surgery and shows you how to find the right doctors to perform them.

Once you have read *Are You Considering Cosmetic Surgery?*, you will be a savvy consumer aware of all the latest trends, including

- why the goal of cosmetic surgery is changing from "reincarnation" to "rejuvenation";
- whether you are better off going to Rio de Janeiro, Miami, or Los Angeles for a surgical makeover;
- the new roles—and controversies—of lasers for cosmetic use;
- the expanding use of endoscopy—operating remotely through tiny incisions—in aesthetic plastic surgery;
- the growing popularity of partial face-lifts such as eyelid- and forehead-lifts;
- whether the World Wide Web is a reliable route to a cosmetic surgeon;
- "facial sculpting" as an alternative to face-lifting;
- why some people become cosmetic surgery junkies;
- whether computer imaging can reliably predict how you will look after surgery;
- why the average age of cosmetic-surgery patients is declining;
- why the proportion of male patients is growing;
- why more cosmetic surgery is being done in doctors' offices and same-day surgical centers instead of hospitals;
- the use of collagen injections to plump up wrinkles

and botulism toxin injections to get rid of scowl lines; and
- why a periodic nip and tuck during your thirties and forties may help you avoid a total face-lift in your fifties or sixties.

Questions about eyebrow-lifts, permanent makeup, cheek and chin implants, double-chin removal, face sanding, chemical peels, laser peels, nose reshaping, ear setbacks, neck-lifts, breast surgeries, cosmetic dentistry, scar revisions, spider-vein removal, thigh-lifts, buttock-lifts, tummy tucks, and liposuction to vacuum out excess fat from the abdomen, hips, thighs, and knees are all explored in the pages that follow.

In some respects, cosmetic surgery is becoming more affordable. According to the American Society of Plastic and Reconstructive Surgeons, 65 percent of people who undergo aesthetic plastic surgery have family incomes under $50,000 a year. There are patients who save up for years or sell mutual funds so they can have cosmetic surgery. Some get it from their husbands as a twentieth anniversary gift. Nurses, secretaries, saleswomen, and teachers drive Toyotas instead of Lexuses because they need the money for their face-lift or liposuction.

After spending $20,000 to have her nose reshaped and her face and eyelids lifted, Heather, a middle-aged teacher from New Jersey, reminded her husband that she needed a new car.

"You're driving your face," he deadpanned.

While doctors' fees have remained high, overall costs have fallen because many procedures formerly done in the hospital are now performed in doctors' offices or same-day surgery centers. How to evaluate a free-standing operating room and where to begin your search for a surgeon are among the important issues examined in Chapter One—must reading for anyone considering cosmetic surgery.

Consumers' need for solid information about cosmetic

surgery has never been greater. Baby-boomers, that demographic landslide of 81 million souls born between 1946 and 1964, didn't have the benefit of sunscreens when they were children. Add the current emphasis on preventive medicine and healthier lifestyles, and you get a huge population of people who look older than they feel. Explains one energetic fifty-seven-year-old two weeks after her face-lift: "I wanted my outside to match how I felt inside."

Mary, who teaches adult education courses, expressed similar sentiments shortly after her full-face laser peel. "I don't mind being fifty," she says, "but I don't want to look fifty."

In addition to witnessing the ravages of time, gravity, and sun exposure on their skin, many boomers are having a hard time shedding layers of fat that are padding their profiles. To make matters worse, they are reminded each time they open a magazine or watch TV that beauty is still defined by a youthful face and lithe body. Dissatisfied with what nature gave them, more and more boomers are starting to fight back.

Their most potent weapon is liposuction, or fat vacuuming. With more than 51,000 patients in 1994 alone, liposuction is now the number one cosmetic procedure in the United States. The number of face-lifts performed annually, meanwhile, leapt 178 percent between 1988 and 1993; the number of eyelid-lifts nearly doubled. According to a 1994 survey of plastic surgeons, 41 percent of all aesthetic surgical procedures were performed on people between ages thirty-five and fifty. Having your forehead, eyelids, cheeks, nose, lips, chin, breasts, belly, thighs, or other body part "done" is becoming almost as socially acceptable as highlighting your hair. Not surprisingly, the stigma of vanity historically associated with cosmetic surgery is vanishing. Industry surveys suggest that the number of people who approve of aesthetic surgery, for themselves or others, has increased 50 percent over the last decade.

Men—particularly middle-aged, white-collar workers

who lost jobs as a result of downsizing and corporate merg-
ers—are also seeking cosmetic surgery in increasing numbers. In 1994, men accounted for 12 percent of aesthetic
plastic surgery patients. When it comes to aesthetic surgery
of the face alone, that statistic jumps to about one in four.
This book is also a valuable resource for parents of children
and teenagers who want cosmetic surgery. An entire chapter is devoted to ear setbacks, male breast reduction, and
other aesthetic procedures typically performed on young
people. Questions about their special emotional concerns
are answered as well.

Having objective, factual information about cosmetic
surgery is vital because nothing short of your health and
well-being are at stake. Patients risk blood loss, infection,
nerve damage, disfigurement, and even death in their quest
for beauty. Results of many cosmetic procedures are temporary. Satisfaction can never be guaranteed. Complications
can arise in the hands of the most skilled surgeons. Clearly,
the decision to have cosmetic surgery should be weighed
carefully. By the time you finish this book, you will know
how to find a qualified plastic surgeon and what to ask
before surgery. You will have a clear idea of which procedure or procedures are most appropriate for you. You will
know what your surgery will cost in money and time. And
most importantly, you will know what to expect—and what
not to expect—before, during, and after your procedure.

❖ 1 ❖

COSMETIC PLASTIC SURGERY

An Overview

CAUSES OF SKIN AGING

Why do I look older than my age?

Blame it on the beach. In pursuit of the perfect tan, you probably soaked in too much sunshine in your childhood and teens. Your skin is now paying the price in the form of dryness, creases, fine lines, wrinkles, brown blotches, and other problems. Research suggests that about 90 percent of skin changes that emerge in your thirties and forties are from exposure to the sun's ultraviolet (UV) radiation. In fact, most wrinkles that form before age fifty can generally be attributed to UV light or cigarette smoking. A study in sunny Queensland, Australia, found that photoaging—the premature aging of chronically exposed skin such as the face and hands—is evident in people as young as twenty-five.

Additionally, UV radiation accelerates the appearance of brown patches, sometimes called "age spots" or "liver spots," which tend to form on older people's faces and hands. Tanning beds are at least as harmful to skin as sunshine.

Why is sunlight so harmful to skin?

UV radiation damages the skin's cellular structure at the DNA level. This microscopic damage builds up for decades before it manifests in wrinkles and other visible skin changes.

Do other factors cause premature aging of the skin?

Yes. Chronic exposure to wind and other outdoor elements hastens skin aging. Just look at a sailor, and the evidence is clear.

Another contributing factor is cyclical weight loss and gain. Yo-yo dieting stretches the skin, causing it to lose its elasticity and making it more vulnerable to wrinkling and sagging under the force of gravity.

Overanimated facial expressions can contribute to wrinkling, albeit to a lesser degree. Smoking also causes premature aging of the skin.

Why does smoking cause wrinkles?

Smoking constricts the small blood vessels in the skin, reducing the oxygen and nutrient supply to delicate facial tissues. Blood-vessel constriction lasts for hours after a cigarette has been snuffed out. Over the years, oxygen and nutrient deficiencies cause skin to lose elasticity, wrinkle, and eventually take on a grayish pallor. Repeatedly pursing your lips to draw on a cigarette accelerates the formation of fine vertical lines around your mouth. Squinting in response to toxins in cigarette smoke causes premature eyelid wrinkling.

What happens during natural skin aging?

A number of things. The epidermis (the skin's outer layer) slowly thins out and loses a portion of its melanin-producing cells. Melanin is a pigment that provides a degree of natural protection from UV radiation. In some older people, melanin collects in clumps, forming age spots.

Also, while the epidermis thins, keratin (the skin's most superficial layer) can thicken and flake off.

More profound changes occur in the dermis, the skin's inner layer. Dermis is comprised mostly of collagen, the strong, fibrous protein responsible for holding all your tissues together. (Leather is almost entirely animal collagen.) As we age, collagen can thin and the skin loses its ability to snap right back after being stretched. Coincident with this process, the normal layer of fat under the skin in areas such as the forearms and cheeks can thin out. While this happens, our genetic program causes pockets of fat to collect in other areas, including the jowls and neck (beneath the chin).

How fast your skin ages is largely determined by your genes, with only the sun, smoking, and poor health as potential contributing factors. For a clue to where your skin is headed without cosmetic surgery, look at your mother or grandmother.

Are all wrinkles the same?

No. There are two kinds of wrinkles: static and dynamic. Static wrinkles are those that are present all the time, even when the facial muscles are at rest. They form in skin that has thinned out and stretched as a result of age. Dynamic wrinkles occur in people of all ages. They form when a muscle contracts and causes the skin overlying that muscle to fold like an accordion. Dynamic wrinkles are present only when the face is animated.

One of the basic principles of facial rejuvenation is that static wrinkles are treatable by a number of methods while dynamic wrinkles are stubborn and would be expected to return soon after any treatment—short of removing the constrictive muscle.

Is the rate of skin aging different for people of color?

Yes. Dark-skinned people have more UV-filtering melanin and are therefore less vulnerable to photoaging. It is not unusual for blacks of African descent to reach their sixties or beyond with barely a wrinkle.

Can cosmetic plastic surgery reverse skin aging, both natural and sun-induced?

Yes and no. Traditional cosmetic surgery such as face-lifts make superficial changes in your appearance by stretching out wrinkles and otherwise manipulating the way your skin forms around your skeletal structure. There are, however, drugs such as Retin-A, possibly topical Vitamin C, and alpha-hydroxy acids that appear to have an anti-aging effect on cells. Under a microscope, skin actually does look younger after treatment with these substances. Similarly, skin that has been chemically peeled or treated with a laser also can look younger. These treatments appear to stimulate the growth of new elastin fibers in the dermis, which enhances the skin's elasticity, or its ability to bounce back after being stretched.

HOW COSMETIC SURGERY CAN HELP

Can cosmetic surgery make me look younger?

Probably. At the very least, it can rejuvenate your appearance and make you look more refreshed. Cosmetic surgery also can make you thinner where you want to be thinner, fuller where you want to be fuller, and improve your profile. Most important, cosmetic plastic surgery can make you feel better about your appearance. That can go a long way toward increasing your self-esteem and your outlook on life.

What exactly is plastic surgery?

Plastic surgery is any operation that repairs, reconstructs, or reshapes the skin and underlying tissue. Procedures to improve your appearance, such as dermabrasion and chemical peels, are informally grouped under the broad category of plastic surgery.

Is plastic used in plastic surgery?

No. The word "plastic" is derived from "plastikos," a Greek word meaning to "mold" or "give form." Thus, plastic surgery molds the human body into a new form.

What is the difference between cosmetic plastic surgery and reconstructive plastic surgery?

Cosmetic plastic surgery, also known as aesthetic surgery, changes the appearance of normal—albeit unattractive or aged—tissue. Reconstructive surgery is done to restore or improve the function of a body part that was disfigured due to injury, birth defect, or disease. It is not unusual for reconstructive surgery to have cosmetic benefits, as well. Cosmetic surgery is labeled "nonessential surgery," meaning your health will not be altered if the procedure is not performed. It also means that in general, medical insurance will not pay the surgeon's fee and related costs. By contrast, "elective surgery" is usually essential but is done on a nonemergency basis. Reconstructive surgery is elective and generally covered by most medical insurance policies. Some operations, such as breast reconstruction following mastectomy, and rhinoplasty (nose reshaping) when done after an accident, are both aesthetic and reconstructive and are often covered. Likewise for deep chemical peels when they are done primarily to remove precancerous skin lesions.

Is cosmetic plastic surgery considered major surgery?

Honest surgeons know that there is no such thing as "minor surgery." Even a simple mole removal (see Chapter Seventeen) may be complicated by infection, scars, bleeding, or an allergic reaction to drugs. Other cosmetic surgical procedures, such as the tummy tuck (see Chapter Fourteen), can last four or more hours and involve a long, uncomfortable recovery period. Cosmetic surgeries carry the same risk factors as essential surgeries, including severe complications such as blood clots traveling to the lungs and even death. Although complication rates are extremely low, their seriousness underscores the importance of thinking things through and investigating the operation thoroughly before making a decision to have cosmetic surgery.

How can I get over my squeamishness about blood, needles, and scalpels?

Most patients are given the option of having their surgery under general anesthesia. Squeamish patients usually prefer to sleep through their operations.

It is also possible to get over your squeamishness during the weeks or months between the time you schedule your procedure and the day of your operation. Heather, the New Jersey teacher, was "really scared of needles" before her face-lift. "But once I decided I was going to have this operation, I had no fear," she relates. "My heart wasn't even pounding when I went into the operating room. I never thought I could be so brave . . . but I was totally determined to have this done."

Empowered by her resolve, Heather was able to conquer her fear.

CHOOSING YOUR DOCTOR

Who performs cosmetic surgery?

Aesthetic plastic surgery is practiced by plastic surgeons as well as doctors in other specialties who have advanced training in cosmetic procedures involving their special areas of expertise. Those include general surgeons, otolaryngologists (also known as head-and-neck or ear, nose, and throat surgeons), neurosurgeons, ophthalmologists, dermatologists, and oral and maxillofacial surgeons.

Be aware that anyone with a medical degree and a license

to practice medicine may legally perform cosmetic surgery in the United States—but that does not mean you should expect your allergist to do a tummy tuck or your obstetrician to perform rhinoplasty.

What certifications should I look for when choosing a cosmetic surgeon?

The most important certification comes from the American Board of Plastic Surgery, one of the twenty-four specialty boards recognized by the American Board of Medical Specialties (ABMS), which sets high standards of education, training, and experience. There are scores of other "self-designated" boards that set their own standards for membership. These standards may incorporate some of the requirements of the recognized surgical specialties. Or they may require nothing but a warm body and a membership fee. (A list of ABMS-recognized boards appears in Appendix A.)

The American Board of Cosmetic Surgery is a self-designated board. Its membership is open to doctors who practice cosmetic surgery but do not necessarily have the qualifications for membership in the American Board of Plastic Surgery.

No matter how prestigious certification seems, it is no guarantee of experience or competence in aesthetic procedures.

What does board certification mean?

Certification by the ABMS-sanctioned American Board of Plastic Surgery means the physician has earned a degree from an accredited medical school and has completed at least three years of supervised general surgical training followed by a two- to three-year residency training program in plastic surgery. Residency training includes both cosmetic and reconstructive surgery. After at least two years of practice, the physician must pass comprehensive written and oral exams in plastic surgery before becoming board certified. This is not a rubber stamp; the failure rate is about 30 percent. Board certification in plastic surgery usually indicates the doctor is trained to do a wide variety of cosmetic procedures on the face and body. Otolaryngologists confine their aesthetic work to the head, face, and neck regions.

Usually, nonplastic surgeons who perform cosmetic surgery concentrate on the part of the body they already specialize in. For instance, a dermatologist might learn to do laser peels to correct facial wrinkles, and an ophthalmologist might seek training in cosmetic eyelid surgery. It is unusual to find a surgeon certified in some other specialty who does general plastic surgery. Likewise, it is unusual to find a general practitioner who is competent performing breast implants. If the doctor has not completed a special surgical residency, be wary.

What kind of training should I look for in a cosmetic surgeon?

Look for an accredited residency program, preferably in plastic surgery. A plastic surgery residency program involves two or three years of training in all cosmetic and reconstructive procedures.

Beyond that, cosmetic surgeons should continually update their knowledge and learn new skills through continuing education courses. This is vital because many state-of-the-art techniques weren't developed or perfected when today's plastic surgeons were in residency programs. The better continuing education courses are sponsored by a professional group such as the American Society of Plastic and Reconstructive Surgeons. Some courses are sponsored by no one except a manufacturer trying to sell doctors a new surgical gadget.

Don't be timid about looking into a doctor's educational background. A doctor's depth and scope of training will probably determine whether you are happy or miserable after your surgery. Prestigious medical schools and residency training programs are highly sought after by doctors, and it is no accident that doctors with excellent credentials are often excellent doctors.

Are there any professional organizations that my surgeon should belong to?

About 97 percent of this country's 5,000-plus board-certified plastic surgeons belong to the American Society of Plastic and Reconstructive Surgeons (ASPRS), head-quartered near Chicago. Only doctors who are board-certified in plastic surgery are permitted to join and become active members. The ASPRS mission includes educating the public about plastic surgery, promoting "high professional standards of care" through its educational foundation, and lobbying government and insurers on behalf of plastic surgeons. Membership in ASPRS, or any professional society, is voluntary.

Another group, the American Academy of Facial Plastic and Reconstruction Surgery (AAFPRS), is primarily for otolaryngologists, the surgeons who specialize in cosmetic and reconstructive procedures of the head and neck. Among other things, this Washington, D.C.–based organization sponsors research, postgraduate training, and continuing education. According to its fact sheet, AAFPRS is dedicated to "maintaining the highest standards for professional and ethical conduct" among its approximately 2,500 members. Not all otolaryngologists practice cosmetic surgery. Only recently have their surgical residency programs incorporated more extensive cosmetic training.

A third association, the American Society for Aesthetic Plastic Surgery, Inc. (ASAPS), based in Arlington Heights, Illinois, requires members to be board certified in plastic surgery and to devote a "significant portion" of their practice to cosmetic procedures. Plastic surgeons must be in practice at least three years before they can apply for membership. In addition to providing information to the public, the aesthetic society's goals include promoting and encouraging the "highest standards of ethical conduct and responsible patient care" among its approximately 1,100 members.

Are hospital privileges important?

Absolutely. In order for doctors to be able to operate in a hospital, they usually must show evidence of proper training, experience, board certification, and expertise. While possessing privileges does not guarantee the person is a good surgeon, *not* having privileges should raise some questions in your mind. Make sure the surgeon you select not only has privileges at a hospital, but that he or she also has privileges to do your particular procedure in that hospital.

Where do I begin my search for a cosmetic plastic surgeon?

There are a number of sources you can tap.

- Your family physician, internist, or gynecologist. Don't take a referral at face value, however. Ask your physician why the cosmetic surgeon is qualified. Your doctor should know the surgeon's reputation through mutual hospital affiliations or other forms of professional contact. A referral is meaningless if your doctor knows the cosmetic surgeon only by his performance on the tennis court or in social situations. Well-meaning family doctors have unwittingly referred patients to unqualified surgeons, according to congressional testimony in 1989 by Harvey Zarem, M.D., a past director of the American Board of Plastic Surgery. A good question to ask your family doctor is "Who would you send your spouse or child to" for rhinoplasty, liposuction, a breast-lift, or whatever procedure you are considering.

- Friends, family members, and acquaintances who have had the same procedure you want. Some questions to ask: How did they find their surgeon? Were they satisfied with the outcome? Would they have done anything differently? Would they use the same surgeon again? How much did the surgery cost?
- An operating room nurse or technician who assists surgeons.
- Your county or state medical society. Medical societies don't recommend one doctor over another, but they can provide a list of board-certified physicians who are members of their organizations. In addition to names and phone numbers, medical societies can tell you which hospitals and medical schools their members are affiliated with.
- *The Marquis Directory of Medical Specialists* (published by Marquis Who's Who) or *The Compendium of Certified Medical Specialists* (published by the American Board of Medical Specialties). Available in most public libraries, these directories list surgeons who are certified by medical boards that are endorsed by the American Board of Medical Specialties.
- A university medical school. Any practicing cosmetic surgeon who also teaches aesthetic plastic surgery has passed an additional layer of scrutiny by his or her peers at the medical school.
- The American Society for Aesthetic Plastic Surgery's toll-free referral service: 1-888-272-7711. This service can provide names of board-certified plastic surgeons in your area who specialize in the kind of cosmetic procedure you want.
- The Plastic Surgery Information Service, 1-800-635-0635. Operated by the American Society of Plastic and Reconstructive Surgeons, this toll-free service can provide names of five board-certified

plastic surgeons in your area. It also can tell you
whether a surgeon you are considering is board certified.
• A hospital physician-referral service. Naturally, a
hospital will refer you to its own doctors. But hospital affiliation implies the doctor meets a certain
level of education, training, and patient care. It further implies that the physician's credentials and
work are subject to review by other doctors. Obtain
referrals only from a major hospital with an impec-
cable reputation.

How many names of doctors should I gather?

Make a preliminary list of three or four qualified candidates. Ideally, you will schedule face-to-face consultations
with at least two before making your final choice. In Appendix B, you will find a "Consultation Comparison
Checklist" that you can photocopy and fill in after each
consultation. The checklist should help you organize your
thoughts and make an "apples-to-apples" comparison.

**Once I have my preliminary list of doctors, what should
I do next?**

If you have not already done so, look up their names in
The Marquis Directory of Medical Specialists or *The Compendium of Certified Medical Specialists* to find out about
their educational backgrounds and certifications.

The doctor's receptionist or nurse may be able to give
you some information over the phone, such as which hospital the doctor uses.

Narrow your list to two finalists for formal consultations,
but retain all your notes. If for any reason you feel uncomfortable with both these doctors, schedule a consultation
with the next qualified surgeon on your list.

WHAT TO EXPECT DURING
YOUR CONSULTATION

What happens during an initial consultation with a cosmetic surgeon?

You and the doctor get to know each other. The doctor listens to your concerns and complaints and performs a physical exam, with an emphasis on the areas of your face or body you want improved. Because the doctor needs to evaluate your skin in its natural state, don't wear any makeup, moisturizer, or other skin-care products to your consultation.

The doctor should ask about your motivations and expectations and discuss how the surgery could affect you psychologically and emotionally. Be totally honest about your feelings. In hopes of obtaining insurance coverage, some patients falsely claim they are seeking to correct a functional problem when their actual goal is strictly cosmetic. If you mislead the doctor about your true motivations for surgery, you could be disappointed with the results. Remember, if you lie in an attempt to have insurance pay for cosmetic surgery, both you and the doctor are committing insurance fraud.

You should be equally forthcoming about your medical history. Tell the doctor about any health problems (medical and psychiatric) and surgeries you've had. Mention any allergies you have and any drugs you are taking—prescription, nonprescription, or illicit. If you smoke cigarettes, be honest about the amount you smoke and how long you've smoked. Smoking, the doctor should warn you, can prolong your healing process and lower the surgery's effectiveness. At the very least, surgeons should advise smokers to avoid cigarettes for several weeks before and after surgery.

You, in turn, must feel free to ask the surgeon anything that's on your mind, including the following.

1. *Do you routinely perform the procedure(s) I want?* There is no hard-and-fast rule about how

many procedures a surgeon must perform monthly or yearly to stay proficient. Ideally, though, your surgeon will have performed your operation hundreds of times. However, with most rarer procedures, such as thigh-lifts (see Chapter Fourteen), or newer procedures, such as endoscopic brow-lifts (see Chapter Two), it may be difficult to find a surgeon with extensive experience. Also remember that even though a surgeon has done a procedure a thousand times, he or she may have done it wrong a thousand times.

2. *What is your favorite procedure to perform?*

3. *Do you enjoy doing the procedure I want?*

4. *Can I talk to any of your patients who had the same surgery?* Most doctors are willing to comply. Of course, you will be referred only to patients who had good results. Still, it can be helpful to speak with someone who has been through the surgery.

5. *Exactly what would happen during my operation?* Even if you've read extensively about your surgery, every surgical experience is unique because every patient is unique. For example, you and your sister may both undergo a face-lift, but your sister may need more skin removed than you do.

6. *Which surgical technique will be used?* As you will see in later chapters, some procedures can be done in a variety of ways.

7. *How long will the procedure take?*

8. *Where will the operation be done?* If it will take place in the doctor's office, ask to see the surgical suite.

9. *Which anesthesia will be used?*

10. *What side effects are associated with the anesthesia?*

11. *How much pain will I experience?*

12. *How long will it be before I can go back to work or be seen in public?*

13. *How long will it take before the full effects of my operation are evident?*

14. *How obvious will it be to others that I had surgery?*

15. *How long will the improvements last?*

16. (If you want surgery on multiple body sites) *Is it possible to do everything in one operation?* This saves you "down time," as long as the surgeon is accomplished in all the procedures. There are, however, additional risks for multiprocedure operations, including increased blood loss and cumulative risks from spending more time under anesthesia.

17. *What is your policy on touchup surgery?* Most doctors will perform revisions in the first year after surgery without a fee. However, there will be fees for use of the operating facility and the anesthesiologist.

18. *What are the risks and complication rates?* The doctor should be extremely forthcoming in response to this important question. Potential risks and complications are listed on the "informed consent agreement" all patients are asked to read and sign before surgery. If the doctor seems reluctant to discuss a procedure's possible downsides, turn around and walk out. To test a surgeon's honesty, ask whether he or she has ever had complications with the procedure. While no doctor likes to talk about this, honest ones will tell you about past complications or worse-than-expected results. The only surgeons who have no complications are those who do not operate—and those who lie.

Do not feel compelled to ask all of the above questions, just the ones that interest you. The purpose of the consultation is to establish a pleasant relationship and get information—not to conduct an inquisition.

You do have a right to expect clear and complete answers to all your questions. Don't be satisfied with an answer that raises other questions in your mind. If the doctor uses a medical term you don't understand, ask for a definition.

It is very important to keep an open mind. Even if you come in requesting a certain procedure, it is the surgeon's job to carefully diagnose the root of your problem and inform you of all your surgical options. For instance, you might have assumed you needed a full face-lift, but your surgeon might suggest an eyelid-lift or laser peel to achieve the results you want. On the other hand, if a doctor recommends a more invasive procedure, listen to your gut instinct. Some doctors actually push a certain procedure because they were recently trained in it or have invested in costly equipment. Likewise, be wary of the surgeon who suggests a procedure unrelated to your concerns. Such behavior is considered unethical by the American Society of Plastic and Reconstructive Surgeons.

You may feel nervous or intimidated during this first consultation. These feelings are fairly typical. It may help to take along a list of questions. After the meeting, jot down your impressions, speak them into a tape recorder, or fill out the checklist in Appendix B.

What if I think of more questions after the consultation?

If you have one or two more questions, the doctor or support staff should be willing to answer them over the phone. Or you can schedule a followup consultation after you've had time to think about everything the doctor told you.

Should I tape record the consultation?

That depends. A tape recorder can be intimidating and limit the free flow of conversation. If you wish to tape your consultation, ask the doctor. Do not take it personally if the doctor says no.

On the other hand, some doctors now record all their consultations. They do this to establish for the medical record that they told the patient about the risks, benefits, and alternatives to treatment, as is required by law.

How much will I be charged for a consultation?

Fees vary regionally and from doctor to doctor. In general, expect to pay anywhere from $100 to $150 or more for a consultation. Some doctors deduct the consultation fee from the surgical fee.

Be very cautious about cosmetic surgery clinics that offer free consultations. These clinics may try to pressure you to sign up for surgery immediately. The adage, "You get what you pay for," couldn't be more true here. These "free" consultations are usually conducted by a nurse, marketer, or secretary, with a five-minute "guest appearance" by the surgeon.

What other factors should I consider before selecting who will do my surgery?

Look for confidence when the doctor explains your procedure. You should feel comfortable discussing your needs, expectations, and any trepidation you might have. Listen to your intuition when evaluating a surgeon's interpersonal style. But don't place too much emphasis on personality. Some doctors are smooth talkers. Don't let a slick presentation overshadow the content of what the doctor says. Be extremely wary of any doctor who *guarantees* satisfaction or an outstanding result.

Here are some more tips offered by the Aesthetic Society.

- Beware of any doctor who tells you there are no possible risks involved in surgery. There are always risks, and these should be discussed frankly.

- Never allow a doctor to talk you into any procedure that you don't want. A reputable plastic surgeon will let patients suggest what they want done and then advise them on what is or is not possible.
- Be skeptical of any doctor who seems to avoid talking about his or her training and professional qualifications.
- Don't "bargain shop" for plastic surgery or fall for gimmicks like rebates, discounts, premiums, gifts, or similar incentives. The training and experience of your surgeon are the most important factors in the success of your surgery.
- Don't compromise.

Finding the right surgeon can be time-consuming, but it is time worth spending because your health, appearance, and self-image are all at stake.

Can I trust a cosmetic surgeon who advertises?

Self-promotion is a controversial issue among medical professionals. Some do it unabashedly; many disdain it. A qualified plastic surgeon who recently relocated to your area may place a modest ad in the newspaper to help build a practice. A less reputable doctor may launch a multimedia advertising campaign that promises miraculous results. If a doctor has enough satisfied customers who are referring their friends and relatives, advertising is not needed. As with other businesses, word-of-mouth is the best form of advertising a doctor can have.

Advertisements in the Yellow Pages are untrustworthy because doctors can promote any procedure they care to sell through the phone book. Likewise, it is difficult to judge a doctor who is quoted in a newspaper or magazine article. On one hand, the doctor could be an authority on cosmetic surgery. On the other hand, the doctor might have hired a public relations specialist to write a press release that caught a journalist's attention.

The latest mode of advertising is the World Wide Web. As of this writing, doctors were being saturated by their professional organizations and marketers to put their faces on the Internet. Most plastic surgery Web sites give brief, superficial descriptions of the procedures a doctor or clinic offers; the fancier Web pages supplement written material with "before" and "after" photos or illustrations. To find current Web sites, search for "cosmetic plastic surgery," or for a procedure you want to know about.

If you discover a cosmetic surgeon through the Internet, newspaper, magazine, or Yellow Pages, investigate his or her background meticulously. Never take an advertisement at face value.

Are unqualified doctors performing cosmetic surgery?

Unfortunately, the answer is yes. Cosmetic surgery in this country is both under-regulated and lucrative—a dangerous combination from the consumer's point of view.

The medical profession as a whole is subject to increasingly strict oversight by cost-conscious health insurers and lawsuit-wary hospitals. Cosmetic surgery has bucked that trend. Cosmetic surgeons get cash up front from patients who pay out-of-pocket. Surgeons often operate in their offices, which, unlike hospital operating rooms, are not required by law to be certified as safe.

With Americans spending billions of dollars each year for surgical beauty enhancement, some doctors who lack extensive training have gotten into the cosmetic surgery business and hung out a shingle. Weeding out the unqualified doctors is not easy. Doctors may actually take weekend courses and then begin performing procedures that others have taken years to learn. It's frightening.

One way to identify a problem doctor is to contact your state's board of medical examiners. These boards are charged with licensing doctors and investigating complaints of professional misconduct. Examining boards also have the power to discipline doctors. Discipline usually takes the form of a reprimand, suspension, or revocation of a medical license, requiring the doctor to complete remedial training, or limiting the scope of a doctor's practice. Action against a doctor's license is public record. The board cannot discuss current investigations or disclose specific complaints against a doctor who has not been formally disciplined.

If actions were taken against a doctor's license in another state, your state board is probably aware of that, according to Dale L. Austin, deputy executive vice president for the Federation of State Medical Boards of United States in Euless, Texas. The federation, to which every medical examining board belongs, operates a national data bank of doctors who have been disciplined. "We encourage our boards to query our data bank when someone applies (for a medical license), and to query the data bank again at the time they are actually ready to give the license," Austin says. "It is that window of time when bad physicians may be trying to jump from state to state." Each month, the federation alerts medical boards of new actions against medical licenses. Boards may take action against a doctor's license based on wrongs committed in other states.

Another organization that keeps track of problem doctors is the Public Citizen Health Research Group, founded by Ralph Nader. Among other things, this nonprofit consumer organization sells a publication called *13,012 Questionable Doctors*, which names physicians who have been disciplined by state medical boards across the country. The publication is helpful only if you want to check specific names since the listings are grouped according to state, not specialty. The three-volume set costs $250 and is purchased primarily by insurance companies and libraries. Consumers can get names of disciplined doctors in their state by sending fifteen dollars to: Public Citizen Health Research Group, 1600 20th Street N.W., Washington, D.C. 20009.

Not all dubious doctors appear in the book. "Sometimes

doctors come in front of the board (of medical examiners), but nothing happens in terms of privileges lost," points out Alana Bame, a consumer specialist at Public Citizen. "They may just get a warning or letter of concern. It's also possible that someone had many of these letters issued, or they had numerous complaints filed against them but did not appear before the panel." Only the "worst offenders" land in *Questionable Doctors*, Ms. Bame notes.

If you have the slightest doubt about a surgeon's competence, find someone else to do the surgery.

PREDICTING SURGICAL RESULTS

How much stake should I put in "before" and "after" photos?

Not too much. First of all, most surgeons will show you only successful cases. Second, no two patients are alike. Even if you have similar age lines as a woman pictured in a "before" shot, your skin type and healing rate can be quite different. Also realize that "before" photographs may be shot in an unflattering light, with the patient frowning and wearing no makeup. The "after" shot may have softer, more flattering lighting, and the patient may be smiling or wearing cosmetics or clothes that enhance her appearance. Remember the photographer's "f-stop face-lift": Open the lens to let in more light, and wrinkles seem to disappear. Different shadows on the "before" and "after" pictures are one clue that the images may have been manipulated by a skilled photographer. Ask doctors if the pictures are of their own patients. Pictures are best used to help you understand the surgery, not to predict your own results. Ask to see photos of "average" results, not "best" results.

Do not be put off if the surgeon declines to show you photographs. Many plastic surgeons feel that photos of successful cases could possibly mislead a new patient.

Can computer imaging show how I'll look after surgery?

New software programs enable a computer to manipulate your current appearance into what you might look like after cosmetic surgery—the key word being "might." Some cosmetic surgeons dislike computer imaging because it can inflate a patient's expectations and imply a guarantee. The last thing a cosmetic surgeon wants is a disappointed patient. Beware of surgeons who use computer imaging as a sales tool to attract new patients or sell you more surgery than you originally intended to have.

Despite its shortcomings, the computer can be helpful for both the plastic surgeon and patient to understand the desired changes and the effects of certain surgical procedures. In rhinoplasty, for instance, the effect of changing the angle between the nose and lip can be readily demonstrated through computer imaging.

"INCISIONLESS" SURGERY

What is endoscopic cosmetic surgery?

Endoscopy—operating remotely through tiny incisions—has been used in knee and abdominal surgery for many years. More recently, the technique has been adapted for certain cosmetic uses.

An endoscope is a tube-shaped probe fitted with a miniature video camera and tiny light. During the operation, an endoscope is inserted under the skin and muscle through an inch-long incision. A picture of internal structures is transmitted onto a television monitor and magnified. Small scalpels, scissors, or forceps are inserted through small nearby incisions and manipulated by the surgeon, who watches the action on the monitor.

The most common cosmetic procedure being done with endoscopes is the forehead-lift. Tummy tucks, breast enlargements, and face-lifts are being done endoscopically on a very limited basis. Endoscopy also may be combined with traditional "open" surgical techniques.

What are the pros and cons of having endoscopic cosmetic surgery?

Endoscopy has several advantages over conventional surgery, which uses longer incisions. Scars are minimal and very easily hidden in the hairline or natural skin fold. Smaller incisions decrease the risk of numb areas after surgery.

There are a number of downsides to consider. Because cosmetic endoscopy is new, it may be difficult finding a surgeon with adequate training and experience. Endoscopy may be more expensive than conventional surgery because it requires expensive instruments. If a surgeon offers to do your surgery endoscopically, ask how many similar endoscopic procedures the doctor has performed and how many hours of training were completed. You don't want to be anyone's guinea pig.

Not everyone is a candidate for endoscopic cosmetic surgery. Cosmetic surgeons tend to prefer to use endoscopes on younger people (thirties and forties) who tend not to have large amounts of loose, hanging skin.

Known risks include infection, fluid accumulation under the skin, damage to blood vessels and nerves, perforation of internal organs, and skin injury, according to the American Society of Plastic and Reconstructive Surgeons. The level of risk depends on the type of surgery being performed. If a problem arises during endoscopy, the surgeon will be forced to complete the procedure through an open incision. Complications occur in about 5 percent of cases, according to the ASPRS.

YOUR HEALTH MATTERS

Are there any medical conditions that would disqualify me for cosmetic surgery?

A poor overall health status—in particular, diabetes, rheumatic diseases, heart disease, lung disease, and certain other chronic conditions—could raise your risk for complications to unacceptable levels. These decisions are made on a case-by-case basis, so it is crucial to give your surgeon a complete and accurate medical history. In some cases, a doctor may suggest a different procedure or a different anesthesia to compensate for your medical condition. Some diseases don't affect your tolerance for surgery but could prolong your healing period or diminish the quality of your results.

Are there any psychological factors that could disqualify me for cosmetic surgery?

Yes, there are several reasons a doctor might refuse to operate on you.

Crisis. As a rule, doctors don't like to operate on people who are experiencing severe emotional strain. If you are mourning the death of your spouse, or you just discovered that your spouse is having an affair with your best friend, it is probably the wrong time for cosmetic surgery. Some patients seek cosmetic surgery as a means of coping with their crisis. A caring physician will tell you to wait until the crisis has passed.

Unrealistic expectations. If you weigh two hundred pounds and hope liposuction can shrink you to a size six, you will only be disappointed. Unless you can tone down your expectations, no trustworthy doctor would take your case. Likewise, it is unrealistic to expect your face-lift or nose reshaping to win back your ex-husband, snare a boyfriend, or get you a promotion. Other examples of unrealistic expectations include looking like your favorite movie star or your twenty-one-year-old daughter.

Pursuit of perfection. If you need a magnifying glass to see a wrinkle you want surgically corrected, the doctor should take pause. No cosmetic procedure is 100 percent effective. If you can't live with the tiniest of physical flaws, no surgical outcome will make you happy. Some perfectionist patients go from surgeon to surgeon until they find someone willing to do their procedures.

Mental illness. An astute plastic surgeon should be able to recognize obvious displays of paranoia, delusions, or other mental illness that could make you a poor surgical candidate. Subtle psychiatric abnormalities are sometimes suspected and should not be taken as an insult if your surgeon requests clearance from a psychiatrist or psychologist prior to surgery. It is for your own protection. If you have a mild depression and suffer a surgical complication, it could send you down a dangerous spiral to severe depression. If you have a diagnosed mental illness, it must be well-controlled for a long period of time prior to any cosmetic procedure.

What are considered appropriate motivations for cosmetic surgery?

The American Society of Plastic and Reconstructive Surgeons has identified two categories of people who make good candidates for cosmetic surgery

1. People with a strong self-image but are bothered by a physical characteristic that they would like to improve or change. "After surgery, these patients feel good about the results and maintain a positive image about themselves," states a ASPRS brochure titled "Psychological Aspects of Plastic Surgery."

2. People who have a physical defect or cosmetic flaw that has diminished their self-esteem over time. "These patients may adjust rather slowly af-

ter surgery, as rebuilding confidence takes time,''
the brochure continues. ''However, as they adjust,
these patients' self-image is strengthened, sometimes dramatically.''

If you want cosmetic surgery to please yourself, not
someone else, then you are on the right track. Studies have
shown that 95 percent of carefully screened cosmetic surgery patients are satisfied with their results.

EVALUATING THE SURGICAL SITE

**Why are 80 percent of cosmetic procedures being done
outside the hospital setting?**

Doctors may emphasize convenience, privacy, and cost-
savings, but the primary reason is insurance. Until several
years ago, some health-insurance policies actually covered
operating-room, anesthesiology, and other hospital expenses even as they rejected claims for cosmetic surgeons'
fees. Depending on where you live, hospital and anesthesiology fees can double the overall cost of your procedure.
Obviously, this development made inpatient cosmetic surgery too costly for many people.

To compensate, plastic surgeons began doing many types
of cosmetic surgery in ambulatory (outpatient) settings, often their own offices. Patients go home the same day as
their surgery, generally a few hours after the anesthesia
wears off.

Hiring a private-duty nurse for your postoperative period
is another cost-cutting option. Private nurses charge around
$400 a night, compared with $2,000 or more for an overnight hospital stay. Some plastic surgeon's offices have the
capacity to keep you overnight under a nurse's supervision,
reducing a lot of postoperative hassles.

What are the advantages of having cosmetic surgery in an ambulatory facility?

Outpatient surgery spares patients the high overhead costs of a hospital operating room and overnight stay. An office-based operating room fee more closely represents expenses incurred, and there is no cost-shifting to a hospital's money-losing programs. In addition, the aesthetics in outpatient facilities are often superior to hospitals. Finally, there are usually more nurses and other support staff per patient in outpatient facilities, particularly in well-run offices.

What are the disadvantages?

The main disadvantage is the lack of regulatory oversight. Unless the ambulatory surgery center is affiliated with a hospital or licensed by the state, neither the center—nor the surgical assistants who work there—have to conform to anyone's standards for patient safety or care. As of this writing, in most states, accreditation of ambulatory surgical facilities outside hospitals and licensed surgicenters is strictly voluntary.

Even if your doctor's surgical suite is clean and has state-of-the-art equipment, you are still at a greater risk if something goes wrong. For example, a woman who suffers a heart attack during her face-lift could be whisked to an emergency room or cardiac unit more quickly if she were in a hospital.

Doctors who do office-based surgery can hire anyone to assist them, although they put themselves at legal risk if the assistant is unqualified. In a hospital, only properly trained and licensed nurses and technicians may assist during surgery. Furthermore, not all office-based operating suites are equipped to administer general anesthesia.

How can I tell whether an office-based operating suite is of high quality?

Make sure your doctor has current hospital privileges. Some doctors operate in their offices because they lost hospital privileges or were unable to get them in the first place. Also, the office-based facility should be dedicated solely to outpatient surgery. It should not be an examination room that doubles as an operating room.

Ask your surgeon if the facility is accredited. A certificate of accreditation should be on the wall. If you don't see it during your presurgery tour, ask where it is. If the doctor cannot produce a current certificate, ask why that is the case. Doctors who invest the energy and money to make their operating facilities worthy of accreditation ought to be delighted to show off their certificates and give patients the grand tour before surgery. The very fact that you asked about accreditation shows you are a savvy consumer who has done her homework.

The main organizations that accredit ambulatory surgical facilities are

- the American Association of Accreditation of Ambulatory Surgery Facilities (AAAASF), (847) 949-6058;
- the Accreditation Association for Ambulatory Health Care (AAAHC), (847) 676-9610; and
- the Joint Commission on Accreditation of Healthcare Organizations (JCAHO), (708) 916-5800.

The American Society of Plastic and Reconstructive Surgeons, (800) 635-0635, maintains a list of accredited outpatient facilities used by its members.

What does an accrediting organization look for before giving its seal of approval?

There are hundreds of so-called "standards" a facility must comply with before being accredited. The standards affect patient care directly or indirectly and address such issues as infection control, anesthesia use, medication use, resuscitation equipment, patient education and patients' rights, data collection, and how the organization discovers and corrects problem areas.

Once a surgical facility is accredited, it must subject itself to periodic on-site inspections to maintain accreditation. A surgeon whose operating room is not accredited may be trying to cut corners. That may be acceptable in a bakery, but not in an operating room.

Why would anyone subject their surgical facility to such an exhaustive inspection process voluntarily?

Free-standing surgicenters run by physician groups are increasingly dependent on managed-care organizations, which often demand accreditation. In the case of cosmetic surgery patients, who choose their own doctors, having an accredited surgical facility is a strong selling point.

While ambulatory surgery continues to be one of the least regulated areas of the medical field, there is a nascent trend in some states toward more regulation. Doctors whose facilities already meet accrediting groups' standards are likely to have an easier time complying with any regulations their state adopts in the future.

For now, do not allow yourself to be placed under general anesthesia in an ambulatory surgical facility unless it is fully accredited.

Is there a difference between a licensed, certified, and accredited facility?

"Licensing" is administered by state departments of health. It involves quality inspections and usually is done only for hospitals and surgicenters. Many states cannot and do not license office operating rooms. That does not necessarily mean these facilities are inferior; it is merely a function of a state's licensing laws.

"Certification" is done by Medicare, the federal health-insurance program for the elderly. Although Medicare has nothing to do with cosmetic surgery, its certification is a measure of quality that is available to qualified office operating rooms, surgicenters, and hospitals where cosmetic surgery is performed. You can generally assume that surgicenters and hospitals have Medicare certification. Most office operating rooms are not Medicare certified because the standards for safety, personnel, record-keeping, and other areas are extremely high. Although Medicare certification is voluntary in most states, the fact that a facility is certified provides a level of assurance to the patient.

''Accreditation,'' performed by one of the aforementioned organizations, is another voluntary, quality-assuring step but, in most states, has no government status.

How can I tell whether a surgeon's assistants are qualified?

Most cosmetic surgeries do not require a true surgical assistant. State laws only require a true ''first assistant'' when a bodily cavity, such as the abdomen or chest, is opened. Most plastic surgeons have scrub nurses or scrub technicians work with them in an office operating room. At least one nurse in an operating or recovery room must be an R.N. (a registered nurse licensed by the state) in all certified or accredited facilities.

A licensed anesthesiologist (M.D.) or nurse anesthetist should be in the operating room if general anesthesia is to be administered. This person should also be on hand for procedures done under local anesthesia coupled with intravenous sedation. If a problem arises during surgery, the patient may need general anesthesia on an emergency basis.

Can anyone have cosmetic surgery as an outpatient?

No. This decision is made on a case-by-case basis. The surgeon must consider your medical history, the length and complexity of your surgery, what kind of anesthesia will be used, and whether someone will be available to drive you home after surgery and help you during your recovery.

PLANNING YOUR SURGERY

Can I drive myself home after the operation?

Absolutely not if you were sedated or given general anesthesia. Even if you only had local anesthesia, you may experience pain or grogginess that could hamper your driving ability. Arrange to have a friend or family member drive you home. Do not call a taxi or limousine. A professional driver should not be given the responsibility of returning you to the doctor if you get sick in the car.

How should I prepare myself for cosmetic surgery?

Although not critical, if possible, do not schedule your surgery during your period because it could increase bleeding. Avoid aspirin, any drugs containing aspirin, and Vitamin E for at least two weeks before surgery because these substances interfere with the blood's clotting action. For similar reasons, avoid ibuprofen and other nonsteroidal anti-inflammatory drugs for forty-eight hours before surgery. Your surgeon will need a list of any medications you take to make sure none hinders the blood's ability to clot. Do not wear makeup on the day of your procedure, and be sure to remove any residual eye makeup. Take a shower before surgery; cleanliness reduces your infection risk. To minimize the possibility of vomiting from medications, do not eat anything for eight hours prior to surgery. This should not be a problem as most surgeries are performed early in the morning. Also, do not wear contact lenses or jewelry into the operating room.

FEELINGS ABOUT COSMETIC SURGERY

Am I vain for wanting cosmetic surgery?

It depends on how you define vanity, and whether you perceive vanity as a negative or positive trait. Are you vain for putting on lipstick and eye shadow every morning, or for wearing clothes without stains or missing buttons? Is it bad to want to look your best? "We all try to improve our self-image in one way or another," Gustavo A. Colon, M.D., president of the American Society of Aesthetic Plastic Surgery, points out. Having cosmetic surgery, he says, is "just another step in the same direction."

Kathy, a twenty-seven-year-old model and actress who had an operation to shave a bump off her nose, views cosmetic surgery as another form of ego-boosting.

"Ego-boosting is always something we need to do ourselves; we can't get it from someone else," she says. "If we feel comfortable about ourselves, nothing can affect our mindset. The better we feel about ourselves, the easier our days are."

I feel guilty for wanting cosmetic surgery. Is this common?

Very. An overwhelming sense of guilt is the number-one problem many patients express during their initial consultation. They think, "If I do this, God is going to punish me." They perceive cosmetic surgery as indulgent, like buying an expensive new car that they don't really need. In most cases, such thoughts are irrational.

Virtually all celebrities are having their bodies contoured, altered, or padded with implants. As a result, American society has grown increasingly tolerant of aesthetic surgery. As long as a doctor, following proper guidelines of ethics and morality, agrees that cosmetic surgery can help you, and as long as your motivations and expectations are appropriate, there is no reason to feel guilty.

If your feelings of guilt persist after discussing them with your doctor, look deep within yourself and do a reality check. Perhaps you want cosmetic surgery to solve some unrelated problem in your life, or maybe you are pursuing a procedure that, in your heart of hearts, you know you don't really need. Hopefully, your doctor will be perceptive and caring enough to refuse to operate under those circumstances. You may feel angry at first. But in the long run, the doctor is probably doing you a favor.

Why do some people get depressed after cosmetic surgery?

Cosmetic surgery involves wounding healthy tissue in order to change your appearance. The sight of stitches, bruises, and bandages where healthy skin used to be can trigger feelings of depression, even regret, in some people. Fortunately for most patients, any negative emotions are short-lived, often dissipating as the healing process progresses and results become visible. Having people to support you emotionally during your recovery can help enormously. If feelings of depression persist for more than a few months, seek help from a mental health professional.

According to Dr. Colon, 90 percent of patients are "happy and excited" after their surgery and do not get depressed. He points out that your risk of postoperative depression is reduced by knowing what to expect during your recovery period.

COSMETIC SURGERY'S CHANGING DEMOGRAPHICS

Why is the average age of cosmetic-surgery patients declining?

Baby boomers, some still in their thirties, are an important emerging market for the plastic surgery community. Some surgeons' organizations have not wasted any time in reaching out to this trend-setting population. Take a colorful brochure published by the Aesthetic Society, titled "Reducing Early Signs of Aging: How Aesthetic Plastic Surgery Can Help Maintain Your Appearance." It includes a checklist of "visible signs of aging" directed at people in their midthirties to early forties. The list includes gradual hooding of upper eyelids, puffiness under the eyes, fine wrinkling around the eyes, finely etched horizontal frown lines in forehead, and localized fat accumulation in the hips, thighs, buttocks, and abdomen. The brochure states: "Having one or more procedures at a younger age may delay the need for more extensive surgery, and many surgeons feel the results may be better both in the short- and long-term."

Why is the proportion of male patients growing?

While the majority of people having cosmetic surgery is female, as many as one in four are male, by some estimates. The high divorce rate and more disposable income provide some explanation. But in recent years, corporate downsizing has probably propelled a significant number of men into the hands of plastic surgeons. Thousands of middle-aged managers earning $100,000 or more a year have found themselves suddenly unemployed and competing for jobs with people half their age. Age discrimination may be illegal in this country, but it still happens, albeit subtly. If cosmetic surgery can slice ten or more years off a man's appearance, age may become a nonissue instead of a deficit in the eyes of some employers.

Why do some people become cosmetic-surgery junkies?

Reasons vary. But one is the enormous pressure in American society to look young and beautiful. Other cultures, such as the Japanese and Native Americans, revere their elders. For them, wrinkles are symbols of experience and wisdom. In America, wrinkles are practically equated with death. And being small-breasted, or God forbid fat, is considered unsexy. The Barbie dolls we used to play with set an unattainable standard for beauty and perfection. So do movie stars, most of whom owe their looks to cosmetic surgeons. Some women won't be satisfied until they look like Barbie or Julia Roberts. For the cosmetic-surgery junkie, every procedure seems to bring out another flaw.

Cosmetic-surgery junkies may be perfectionists in other areas of life, as well. They are never satisfied no matter how many procedures they get. A psychological evaluation may be warranted in such cases. If a plastic surgeon wisely refuses to indulge a junkie's request for more and more procedures, there is no stopping her from finding another surgeon—as long as her checkbook holds out.

Not everyone who has numerous cosmetic procedures is compulsive, mind you. Some simply enjoy the emotional "lift" cosmetic surgery can give them, and they can afford to indulge themselves.

What can I do to prolong the effects of my surgery?

If you are a sun worshiper, buy a beach umbrella, and use sunscreens with SPF 15 or greater whenever you venture out of doors during the day for more than twenty minutes. Any steps you take now to reduce your UV light exposure will slow down your skin's aging process—and reduce your risk of skin cancer. Sun exposure in the first six months after surgery will cause your incision scars to stain brown.

Smoking cessation will go a long way toward keeping a youthful appearance, as will minimizing your alcohol consumption.

TRAVELING FOR COSMETIC SURGERY

Why have Rio and Buenos Aires become such popular destinations for cosmetic surgery?

Marketing, politics, and thong bikinis. Cosmetic surgery clinics in these image-conscious cities have invested heavily in public relations and advertising to attract foreign clientele. CNN, numerous women's magazines, and influential newspapers, including the *Wall Street Journal* and the *Christian Science Monitor*, have responded by running feature stories on the cosmetic surgery surge in Rio and Buenos Aires. According to the *Wall Street Journal*, as many as 240,000 Argentines—in a country of 33 million—underwent cosmetic surgery in 1996.

Widespread interest in cosmetic surgery reportedly took off in Argentina when President Carlos Menem was elected in 1989. Menem, an avid partygoer who has posed for photo shoots with celebrities like supermodel Claudia Schiffer, had surgery to fill in his receding hairline. His estranged wife, Zulema Yoma, "has had so many operations her smile is virtually fixed in place," the *Journal* reported in February 1996. That same year, a book about Argentina's cosmetic surgery craze, titled *The Masks of Argentina*, was a bestseller.

Rio is home to several plastic surgeons with international reputations, including one who boasted to a magazine reporter, "We're the best in the world." That air of confidence has helped draw royalty, celebrities, and socialites to Rio's luxurious clinics. Some cosmetic surgery clinics go so far as providing patients with limousine rides from the airport and five-star hotels to recuperate in. One of Rio's newest trends is having a total surgical makeover—including a face-lift, liposuction, breast reduction, and tummy tuck—in one fell swoop.

Because the cosmetic surgeons in Brazil and Argentina do so many procedures, you might think that their skills are indeed the best in the world. But there is no evidence that their results are any better than those obtained by qualified plastic surgeons in the United States. One prominent South American surgeon reportedly selects patients based on nude photographs without meeting or examining them first.

It can be difficult if not impossible to investigate the

credentials of a doctor who practices abroad. Every country sets its own medical education and certification requirements, and every country has its own standards of patient care. In Argentina, for example, the Argentine Society of Plastic Surgeons has 150 members. But there are at least another two hundred Argentines practicing plastic surgery who are not members of the society, according to a recent report in the *Christian Science Monitor*.

The language barrier is another potential problem. If you don't speak Spanish or Portuguese and your doctor and nurses are less than fluent in English, you may be unable to convey something important about your health status or medical history. Should a mistake be made during surgery, it can be extraordinarily difficult to sue for malpractice in a foreign country.

Despite the potential for problems, going to Rio or Buenos Aires for plastic surgery has become a status symbol in some American social circles. Other Americans are motivated by price. The fees charged by South American cosmetic surgeons are roughly half of their American counterparts. Of course, some or all of that savings is offset by travel, meal, and lodging expenses. Remember that some cost savings may be at the expense of safety.

Before deciding to have surgery in a foreign country, find out as much as you can about the doctor and the clinic by talking with former patients and studying the doctor's curricula vitae. Question the doctor just as you would question an American doctor before deciding whether to place yourself under his or her care.

What about Miami, Los Angeles, and New York City? Aren't those cities famous for plastic surgery?

The large elderly population in Miami and the concentration of bodies beautiful in L.A. keep the cosmetic surgeons in those cities very busy. Unless you have evidence that a surgeon is sufficiently trained to do your procedure, protect yourself by going through the same investigative process described earlier in this chapter. In the case of New York, having an office on Park Avenue means nothing more than the doctor leased an office on Park Avenue.

SMOOTHING THAT FURROWED BROW

Forehead/Brow-Lifts

My face looks sad and tired even when I am happy and alert. Some people have even said I look angry when I am not. What is happening?

Your forehead is probably showing its age. As with all tissue, the tissue of the forehead stretches out and loses elasticity as we get older. This can cause your eyebrows to descend, crowding your upper eyelids. Sagging eyebrows can make eyelid skin droop over your eyes, creating that tired or stern appearance.

Any aging of the forehead is noticeable relatively early in life, even in the late thirties. This is because the position of the eyebrows, as they relate to the eyes, is apparent if there is a drop of as little as two millimeters. Over time, horizontal expression lines that once displayed themselves only on your command get deeper and remain visible when your forehead is relaxed. Fine wrinkles eventually become deep crags. The lax skin and underlying tissues can no longer hold your eyebrows in their natural position. This often leads to an almost constant spasm of the forehead muscle in order to let in maximal light to your eyes.

Another possible cause of forehead creases is overactive forehead muscles. Overactive facial muscles contract in-

44

voluntarily, creating creases that eventually become permanent.

I have deep lines between my eyebrows, which make me look angry. What causes this?

Frown lines, or "scowl lines," those deep vertical creases between the eyebrows, are caused by overactive muscles known as "corrugator" muscles. Normally, frown lines are visible only in certain facial expressions. Permanent frown lines are usually inherited. They can be prominent in people as young as twenty-five.

How can I tell if a forehead-lift would improve my appearance?

Go to a mirror and examine your forehead. Now raise your eyebrows as high as you can and notice where the horizontal creases are. Now completely relax your forehead muscles. Are any creases or lines still there? Look at a photograph of yourself taken fifteen or more years ago. Notice the position of your eyebrows relative to your upper eyelids. Look in the mirror again. Do your eyebrows sit lower on your face? Do your eyes look smaller? Do the tips of your upper eyelashes touch the bottoms of your eyebrows? Is there hooding of skin over your eyes? If you answer yes to any of these questions, you might benefit from a forehead-lift, also known as a brow-lift. If the rest of your face still looks good, a brow-lift alone would probably suffice. More commonly a brow-lift is performed along with eyelid surgery (see Chapter Three) or a face-lift (see Chapter Four).

Are there cultural differences in what an attractive brow should look like?

Yes. South American women, for example, tend to favor higher eyebrows, up to three-quarters of an inch above the bony "orbital rim" of the eye socket. This position may give you a permanent "surprised" look, so be careful.

There are also changing trends in what is considered aesthetically pleasing. Brow-lifts performed in the 1960s resulted in a high-arching eyebrows (a la Phyllis Diller). Today in the United States, at least, a lower, more natural eyebrow is in favor. Nonetheless, there may be significant differences of opinion between what you and your plastic surgeon consider aesthetically pleasing. Be sure to discuss eyebrow height and arch with your doctor before surgery.

What will I look like after a forehead-lift?

To get a general idea, place your fingers across your hairline and gently pull your forehead skin back so the creases smooth out and your eyebrows raise slightly. The ideal position of the eyebrow should be at the level of the bony orbital rim close to the nose, rising gently to just above the rim as they go toward your ears.

What is the purpose of a forehead-lift?

The forehead-lift is designed to smooth out forehead furrows, lift sagging eyebrows, and, if necessary, minimize scowl lines between the eyebrows. Indirectly, the forehead-lift may reduce some wrinkling in the upper eyelid. Like most types of aesthetic facial surgery, the operation is designed to rejuvenate your appearance.

What are the limitations of this surgery?

A forehead-lift will not reduce puffiness around the eyes, especially beneath the lower eyelids. It also has no effect on the lower two-thirds of the face. It is less effective at reducing horizontal wrinkles and lines than it is in reducing the scowl lines between the eyebrows.

How many surgical options are there for the forehead-lift?

There are two possible approaches: the traditional "open-incision" surgery and the newer "closed" endoscopic technique, where the surgeon operates remotely through small incisions. In some cases, both methods are used to achieve the desired result.

How does the surgeon decide which method to use?

If the surgeon is not trained in endoscopy, there is no decision to make. If there is a choice, several factors must be considered, including the patient's age, forehead height and curvature, depth and number of furrows, skin elasticity, and amount of excess forehead skin. Surgeons prefer to use endoscopy on younger patients—those under age forty-five who do not have redundant (excess) skin. The traditional "open" surgery is preferred for older patients who need excess skin and muscle removed. The chief advantage of the endoscopic brow-lift is that it eliminates a long scar within the hair. This is important because there will be hair loss on the scar, and the skin behind it will always have some degree of numbness. The chief disadvantage of the endoscopic technique is that it is so new that the long-term results, compared to the traditional brow-lift, have not been assessed.

What kind of anesthesia is used during the traditional operation?

Most patients prefer a general anesthesia so they can sleep through the procedure. The operation also can be done under local anesthesia, whereby the patient is sedated and the forehead and scalp injected with a numbing medication.

Regardless of the type of anesthesia used, you will probably have an intravenous line placed in your arm as a safety precaution. This allows medication to be delivered quickly, if necessary.

Where are traditional brow-lifts usually performed?

This operation can be done in a hospital or ambulatory surgical facility. If general anesthesia is to be used, surgeons may prefer to operate in a hospital, even if you are to go home the same day. Any non-hospital-based facility where general anesthesia is used must be extremely well equipped to accommodate an anesthesiologist. If you are to be placed under general anesthesia outside a hospital setting, make sure the surgical facility is fully accredited (see Chapter One).

How should I prepare for the traditional forehead-lift?

Wash your hair the morning of surgery. Do not eat, and take only medications approved by your surgeon. To reduce the risk of infection, you will wear a hospital gown during the operation.

How will I be prepared for surgery?

You may be given a sedative such as Valium a couple of hours prior to surgery. The surgeon or an assistant may tie your bangs into a series of tiny ponytails held with sterile rubber bands in order to expose the area of the scalp to be cut. Or your hair may be simply combed in such a way as to expose the incision area. A half-inch-thick strip of hair is then shaved because the surgeon won't want to cut through hair. A topical germ-killing solution is applied to the area. Local or general anesthesia is then administered.

Where is the incision made?

In a traditional lift, the surgeon uses a scalpel to make an incision across the scalp, from the top of one ear to the top of the other. The incision can be just below the hairline or up to four inches inside the hairline. Where to cut usually depends on the natural height of the patient's forehead. If someone has a long, high, curved forehead, the incision should probably fall just in front of the hairline. Cutting behind the hairline lengthens the forehead by one-quarter to one-half inch. Some women compensate by changing their hairstyles. Bald men are not generally candidates for this operation because the scars would be too difficult to hide.

The incision goes through the thin sheet of forehead muscle but does not cut through a deeper layer of tissue called the periosteum, which covers the skull and other bones. The periosteum is, however, penetrated closer to the eyebrows.

What happens next?

The surgeon peels back the forehead skin and muscle down to the top of the eyebrows. While doing this, the surgeon may thin out any overactive muscles by cutting through some muscle fibers. Most often, the corrugator muscles are cut to eliminate scowl lines. Enough muscle must be left intact for facial expressions, although most surgeons do completely obliterate the scowl muscles. The removal of the corrugator muscle is very precise in order to avoid creating a depression between the brows. Sometimes "filler" material, such as connective tissue or fat (see Chapter Eight) is placed under the skin to fill a depression. The surgeon is careful to avoid cutting or damaging the nerves, which supply sensation to the forehead. If nerves do get cut or stretched during surgery, you may experience numbness, tingling, and itchiness for several months following surgery.

The surgeon then cuts away a strip of skin from the top of the forehead. The amount of tissue removed depends on how much excess skin you have. Removing a strip one-half to three-quarters of an inch wide is typical.

The surgeon then pulls the remaining forehead skin and muscle back up, introducing enough tension to smooth out crease lines. The wound is closed with sutures or surgical staples. Some surgeons use two layers of sutures, dissolvable ones underneath and temporary ones outside.

The incision site is dressed with antibiotic ointment and bandaged with sterile gauze.

How long does the traditional forehead-lift take?

This procedure lasts two to two and a half hours, in most cases. Surgery that combines a forehead-lift with a face-lift takes about five hours.

How bloody is the traditional forehead-lift?

There should be minimal bleeding with this operation.

How is bleeding controlled?

Surgeons can use special clamps, sutures, or electroco-agulation, which heat-seals blood vessels with a high-frequency electrical current. If the scalpel is equipped to deliver this electrical current, virtually bloodless incisions are possible, but there would be more hair loss with this technique.

How much hair will I lose?

If the incision is made inside the hairline, you probably will not lose more than a half-inch of hair-bearing scalp. The goal, however, is to have *no* hair loss.

How can I hide the scar?

Makeup or bangs can mask a scar in front of the hairline. Scars inside the hairline are easily covered by hair, although hair will not grow in the scar itself.

What will I feel immediately after surgery?

You will probably have a headache, although the incision area itself is usually more numb than painful. Twenty to 30 percent of people experience nausea after surgery despite the doctor's best attempts at avoiding drugs that cause nausea and using drugs to treat it.

Your face will most likely swell up, and your eyelids will be black and blue. The swelling may cause temporary blurred vision.

What can I take to control the pain after I get home?

Acetaminophen with codeine or oxycodone is usually needed the evening after surgery and the next day. After that, any pain usually can be controlled with plain aceta-minophen. Avoid aspirin and other nonsteroids, such as ibuprofen, because they can make you bleed for up to two weeks following surgery.

When can I wash my hair?

Most surgeons have patients begin showers and shampoos two days after surgery, after the bandages come off. Use baby shampoo, which causes the least damage to unhealed skin.

When do my stitches come out?

About seven to fourteen days after surgery. The removal process is not painful because the incision site is still a little numb.

What complications are possible after surgery?

One is a hematoma—localized bleeding or blood clot under the skin. Depending on the amount of blood involved, a hematoma can range in seriousness from minor to one that can destroy skin. Small hematomas usually disappear on their own. Bigger ones may need to be drained with a syringe and needle by your surgeon.

Another potential problem is nerve damage. Damaged nerves in the forehead can result in a temporary or permanent loss of sensation, localized loss of muscle movement, or both. Any paralysis usually disappears in time as you retrain your muscles for facial expression.

Recurrence of forehead lines is not really considered a complication. Some horizontal lines will return as swelling decreases, but probably not to the extent seen before surgery. The main reason lines don't return completely is because once the brow is surgically lifted, the brain no longer sends the message to the forehead muscles to raise the brow to let in more light to the eyes. You could also see a return of scowl lines, although this is less likely.

When will I be able to go out in public?

The recovery period is usually ten days to two weeks, but you can go out sooner if you cover your bruises with makeup or wear bangs.

Some people develop black-and-blue marks down to the middle of the face or to the lower face because blood seeps down under the force of gravity. Extensive bruising is more likely to occur if your forehead lift was combined with a face-lift. You can cover bruises with makeup specifically designed for that purpose. Dermablend and Physician's Formula are two excellent brands.

How much does a traditional forehead-lift cost?

Surgeons' fees range from $1,500 to $5,000, with the national average being about $2,000. In general, fees do not include anesthesia, operating room costs, and related expenses, which can add more than $1,000 to the total.

How long will my forehead-lift last?

Most people see a return of furrowing and a descent of the brow in five to ten years. A few patients have problems again in two years. If muscle has been removed to prevent scowling, this change should be permanent.

Can I have a second forehead-lift?

It is possible, but requests for a repeat forehead-lift are very rare.

What happens during an endoscopic forehead-lift?

The surgeon makes three to five cuts just behind the hairline through which the endoscope and other surgical tools will be inserted. Each cut goes clear through to the skull to lift the periosteum (the connective tissue covering the bone), muscle, and skin from their bony attachments. The corrugator muscle fibers are removed to minimize creases and scowl lines caused by overactive muscles. The surgeon then raises the muscle and skin upward and fixes the tissue to a higher level. There are a variety of fixation methods available to the surgeon. Some use small screws into the skull, which are removed in a week. Other methods use sutures. Fixation of the brow is one aspect of this new operation that still has not been perfected.

What are the advantages of endoscopic forehead-lift?

Endoscopy does not elongate the forehead. It leaves just a few small scars hidden inside the hairline compared with the ear-to-ear scar left by a traditional forehead-lift.

Smaller incisions reduce the areas of numbness in the scalp after surgery. There is also less hair loss.

Endoscopy appears particularly well-suited to correct scowl lines. One study of eighteen patients aged twenty-six to fifty who had endoscopy found that corrugator muscle function was reduced by an average of 65 percent seven months postoperatively. The patients' scowl lines were still visible, but they were not as deep as before the operation, according to Dr. Robert S. Hamas, the Dallas plastic surgeon who conducted the study. "The patients were especially pleased that the scowling look they previously had was eliminated."

What are the downsides of the endoscopic forehead-lift?

The technique is so new that it can be difficult to find a surgeon with adequate training and experience. Even when performed by the most skilled hands, the endoscopic forehead-lift presents a higher chance of injury to sensory nerves or nerves that control the forehead and eyelid muscles. There are little data on long-term success and complication rates. According to the American Society of Plastic and Reconstructive Surgeons, known complications include infection, fluid accumulation under the skin, damage to blood vessels and nerves, and skin injury. If a problem arises during endoscopy, the surgeon will be forced to complete the procedure through an open incision. Complications occur in about 5 percent of cases.

Because skin is not removed to tighten the forehead, there is considerably more postoperative swelling under the skin compared with the open technique. Some patients report that their faces continued to swell up in the morning six weeks after the operation.

Until the surgeon hones his or her skills, endoscopy can take longer than the open forehead-lift. Endoscopy also tends to be more expensive because the surgeon has invested in endoscopic instruments, which can cost upwards of $25,000.

Not everyone is a candidate for endoscopic forehead-lifts. Doctors prefer to operate on younger people (thirties and forties) who do not have large amounts of loose, hanging skin. While endoscopy can effectively lift sagging skin, it does not facilitate the cutting away of excess skin and muscle.

What is the cost of an endoscopic forehead-lift?

Generally, this surgery costs about the same as a traditional forehead-lift, although some surgeons may add a little premium to help pay for the specialized equipment involved.

Is there a nonsurgical way to get rid of scowl lines?

Yes, but it is risky. The method involves paralyzing the overactive corrugator muscles with injections of botulinum toxin. Botulinum toxin is derived from the bacteria that causes botulism, a serious food-borne illness. The paralysis is temporary. After four to six months, paralysis subsides and scowl lines return unless another injection is administered.

While the initial injection effectively minimizes scowl lines, subsequent injections appear to be less effective, possibly because the body makes antibodies that destroy the toxin. Another problem is a dearth of research into the toxin's long-term safety. No one knows, for example, whether repeated exposure to botulinum toxin will eventually kill the muscle. Some physicians refuse to administer the injections for that reason. The more "holistic" plastic surgeons worry about the very idea of injecting toxins into the body. These injections should probably be reserved for people who have tics, or uncontrolled muscle spasms in their facial or eyelid muscles.

Each injection costs up to $800.

❖ 3 ❖

THE EYES HAVE IT

Eyelid Surgery

Why is cosmetic surgery of the eyelids so popular?

As a great philosopher once said, the eyes are the windows to the soul. They can also be the windows to our age. Upper eyelids generally begin to sag by your third decade, although some teens already have extra fat and skin on their upper lids. In your forties, the sagging can worsen, and eyelid wrinkles can begin to form. Meanwhile, puffy "bags" may emerge under your lower lids. These changes make your eyes look smaller, your face look older, and cause you to project an image of chronic fatigue.

Successful eyelid surgery, also known as blepharoplasty or eyelid-lift, can rejuvenate your whole face by tightening and restoring contour to droopy eyelids and eliminating the bags. After surgery, your eyes seem bigger and brighter, which gives you a more alert, youthful appearance. Enough Americans have discovered this to make blepharoplasty this country's second most popular facial cosmetic procedure. Among Asian women, blepharoplasty ranks number one because it gives their eyes a more Western look.

Why do my upper eyelids sag?

Over time, the eyelid skin thins and becomes increasingly susceptible to the force of gravity. In addition, the muscle responsible for elevating the eyelid can become stretched, causing the lid's natural position to drop. As a result, the upper eyelids sag and may eventually cause hooding over the eyes.

Hooded eyelids are not necessarily age-related. Joan, an independent consultant from Pennsylvania, was just forty years old when she underwent her blepharoplasty.

"My eyelids, genetically, were very heavy, particularly on one side," says Joan, a mother of two. "Because I lead such an active life, my eyes felt so tired at end of day—more tired than I could afford to be." The operation, she says, corrected her problem and made applying makeup more enjoyable.

Can hooded eyelids obstruct vision?

Yes. Severe hooding of the upper eyelids can obstruct peripheral vision and reduce your range of upward vision. If your plastic surgeon or ophthalmologist makes this diagnosis, your health-insurance policy may cover blepharoplasty because it restores a normal visual field by eliminating the hoods. Be sure to get written confirmation of reimbursement from your insurance company before going ahead with the surgery if finances are a concern.

Why do I have bags under my eyes?

This can have one or more causes. The first is changes in the "orbital septum," a membrane that holds in place a series of fat pads that protect the eye within the eye socket by flotation. If the orbital septum weakens due to age or heredity, the fat protrudes, forming bags or pouches beneath the lower lids.

The second factor is thickening of the eye muscles, which can create the appearance of bags.

Bags also may be a symptom of certain medical conditions, such as thyroid and kidney disease. If they are not already diagnosed, these disorders should be considered before eyelid surgery is performed.

What if my medical condition is being treated, but the bags under my eyes won't go away?

Then eyelid surgery can be used to correct the cosmetic symptoms of the disorder.

Can cosmetic surgery get rid of the dark circles under my eyes?

It depends. If the circles are actually shadows cast by sagging lower eyelids, a lower eyelid-lift can correct the problem.

If the circles are dark pigmentation of the skin, your options are using skin-bleaching creams containing hydroquinones, or a light chemical skin peel using trichloracetic acid, or TCA (see Chapter Six). Bleaching cream must be applied twice daily for several months before an improvement can be seen. The TCA peel yields improvement in a few days.

Circles also may stem from very thin, translucent skin. In this situation, the reddish/purplish hue is caused by blood vessels and muscle just below the skin. The only remedy here is to hide your dark circles with makeup.

A careful examination by a plastic surgeon can usually pinpoint the source of the dark circles.

Can eyelid surgery get rid of my "crow's feet"?

Eyelid surgery is not effective against crow's feet, also known as laugh lines. These "dynamic wrinkles" at the outer corners of the eyes are produced by contraction of underlying muscle—as opposed to wrinkles that form on sagging skin.

Laser peels (see Chapter Seven) and chemical peels (see Chapter Six) can lessen crow's feet to a certain extent.

Will I need an eye exam before my operation?

Some plastic surgeons insist that patients undergo a thorough eye examination, including glaucoma testing, by an ophthalmologist prior to surgery. The exam should also include measurements of teardrop production. If a patient is diagnosed with dry eyes, it could complicate the healing period and necessitate a procedure that tightens the lower eyelid horizontally. If the dry-eye condition is very severe, some plastic surgeons will refuse to perform blepharoplasty. Dry eye problems combined with eyelid skin removal can result in injury and infection of the cornea after surgery.

How old is the average blepharoplasty patient?

There are two age groups that typically seek eyelid surgery. The first are people who develop excess skin and fat on their eyelids in their teens or childhood. This population usually has the surgery in their early twenties. The second group experiences eyelid changes as a result of aging; they start coming in for surgery in their midthirties. Eyelid surgery continues to be sought by people all the way into their seventies, even their eighties.

Can eyelid surgery be combined with a brow-lift or face-lift?

Yes. In fact, the surgeon should consider the position and laxity of your brow when evaluating you for an eyelid lift. If the brow is too lax, a lid-lift can actually drag the brow down farther, making blepharoplasty practically useless. In some cases, it might appear that the upper lids are sagging because there is too much skin when the real problem is a sagging brow. If both the brow and lids are too lax, the best solution is having a combination brow-lift and eyelid-lift. Proper diagnosis is critical to a satisfactory result.

Even more common is having eyelid surgery in conjunction with a face-lift since a face-lift alone will not affect the appearance of the lids. The advantage to having multiple procedures in one operation is a shorter recovery period and less "down time" because your bruises and incisions heal simultaneously. The disadvantage is an increased risk of complications such as bleeding, and having to endure a longer operation—up to six hours for a combined procedure. Patients under local anesthesia tend to get antsy and lose their ability to cooperate with the surgeon when an operation lasts more than a couple of hours.

Is blepharoplasty a particularly difficult operation to perform?

Blepharoplasty—"bleph" is derived from the Latin word for "eyelid"—is an extremely delicate procedure that must be done exceedingly carefully by a well-trained, experienced surgeon. If your procedure is mishandled, you can lose your sight. This rare complication occurs in 4 in 10,000 patients.

What can happen to make a patient go blind?

Fat that is removed during a blepharoplasty is connected with all the other fat pads surrounding the eye. This means that blood can collect behind the eyeball if bleeding of the fat occurs during or after surgery. The simple act of bending down or vomiting can trigger bleeding within the first few hours after blepharoplasty. Symptoms would include intense pain and blurred or lost vision. If not treated rapidly, permanent blindness can result. For this reason, patients must stay in the recovery room a minimum of two hours after the operation. They should remain as quiet and still as possible over the next twenty-four hours.

Is it better to have a general plastic surgeon, an ear, nose, and throat surgeon, or an ophthalmologist do my eyelid surgery?

Generally, cosmetic eyelid surgery is performed by plastic surgeons. Some ophthalmologists are trained in blepharoplasty and have excellent results. Consumers should recognize, however, that the bulk of an ophthalmologist's practice is restoring or improving function of the eyeball and surrounding tissue. Plastic surgeons, by contrast, are oriented more toward aesthetics.

If you are considering an ear, nose, and throat surgeon (otolaryngologist), find out which board certification the physician holds. Follow the guidelines set forth in Chapter One to ascertain whether the surgeon has the proper credentials and training to perform blepharoplasty.

Where is eyelid surgery performed?

Ninety-nine percent of the time, blepharoplasty is performed in an office-based operating room or other outpatient facility. A hospital stay is not usually necessary, as long as the patient has someone to drive her home and help out during the next few days.

How long does the procedure take?

If you are having both upper and lower eyelids done, the operation usually lasts two to two and a half hours. If surgery is being performed on just the upper or lower lids, the procedure takes about one hour and fifteen minutes.

What kind of anesthesia is used?

Blepharoplasty can be done under local anesthesia with sedation, or under general anesthesia. Most patients who opt to have local anesthesia with no sedation later say that they wish they had been sedated during the operation. Modern sedatives such as midazolam or propofol are extremely short-acting and allow rapid recovery prior to going home.

If I am awake during the operation, what will I experience?

You will feel no pain since the area being operated on is numbed. You will see nothing because steel contact lenses are protecting your eyes. You may smell smoke as the surgeon's electrocautery device heat-seals blood vessels. The main thing you will hear is conversation of the operating team, and perhaps music in the background.

How will the surgical team prepare me for the operation?

You will be given a hospital gown to wear and will have to remove all your clothing except for your underwear. This is the routine for most cosmetic surgeries. Sticky pad electrodes will be placed on your chest to monitor your heart's electrical activity (EKG) during surgery. A cuff will be placed on your arm to monitor your blood pressure, and a plastic oxygen monitor will be placed on your finger.

While you are in a sitting position, the surgeon will place marks on your upper and lower eyelids corresponding to the fat pads and extra skin that is to be removed. An intravenous line will be placed in your arm to administer medications during the operation. An antiseptic solution will be applied to your face to sterilize the area, and sterile drapes will be placed around your eyes. Your eyes will be anesthetized with eye drops and steel contact lenses will then be placed in your eyes to protect them during surgery. The anesthetic, lidocaine, will be injected through a thin needle into the areas around your eyes. If you are to sleep through the operation, general anesthesia is administered and a breathing tube is placed through your mouth into your trachea (windpipe).

What happens during the procedure?

The surgeon makes an elliptical incision in the crease of the upper eyelid. Excess skin is removed, exposing the underlying muscle. A strip of muscle several millimeters thick is then removed to help define the eyelid crease after surgery. The surgeon then penetrates the orbital septum to expose three fat pads. A small amount of fat is removed from each pad. The surgeon may either close the incision immediately before turning to the next eye, or the incision may be left open while the second eye is being operated on. Some surgeons prefer the latter approach because it gives them more time to check for bleeding before repairing the wound. The wounds are closed with a single layer of sutures.

There are two currently acceptable methods of lower eyelid blepharoplasty, which is geared toward removing bags and tightening the lower eyelids. The traditional approach requires an incision just below the lower lashes, exactly where eyeliner goes. The surgeon lifts the skin and muscle to expose two fat pads and removes a small amount of fat. Excess skin and muscle are then trimmed from the lower lid, and the wound is stitched closed.

If there is protruding fat but no excess skin, then a so-called "incisionless" blepharoplasty can be done. In actuality there is an incision; it's just hidden inside the lower eyelid. Through this hidden incision, the surgeon exposes the fat pads and trims them. The wound is left to heal naturally because stitches would be too irritating to the eye. This procedure, called the "transconjunctival blepharoplasty," has gained popularity over the last several years.

What other risks are associated with blepharoplasty?

There is a tiny risk of infection, generally less than 1 percent. There is a similar risk of bleeding severe enough to require more surgery. The risk of the scar being visible is minimal.

If the surgeon removes too much skin underneath the eye or there is excessive scarring inside the lower lid, the patient may develop an "ectropion"—a pulling down of the lower lid, creating a basset-hound appearance. An ectropion may be temporary, disappearing as the swelling goes down. If the condition persists, the patient may require corrective surgery.

A good surgeon will recognize which patients are most likely to develop an ectropion and perform a lid-tightening procedure to prevent it. This procedure, known as a "canthopexy," involves shortening the lower eyelid's horizontal length. It is analogous to tightening your belt so you can tug down on your pant legs to smooth out the wrinkles without pulling your pants down. Ten to 20 percent of blepharoplasty patients require a canthopexy. The procedure has the additional benefit of improving the flow of tears through the duct system.

How much pain will there be after surgery, and how can I control it?

Patients report a burning type of pain of mild to moderate intensity. You will probably need codeine the evening after surgery and perhaps the next day. After that, you may need acetaminophen or nothing at all. Placing ice packs on the eyes relieves pain and discomfort and reduces swelling in the first twenty-four hours following surgery.

What else can be done to lessen postoperative swelling?

Some surgeons prescribe intravenous steroids in the recovery room, but this is of questionable benefit.

Keeping your head elevated for several days is of paramount importance. This means sleeping in an easy chair, if possible, sleeping in bed with a booster behind you, or laying your head on two pillows or a U-shaped travel pillow.

Do not, under any circumstances, lie face down during the first two to three weeks after surgery. This can be difficult to do. It may help if, for five minutes before going to sleep each night, you try repeating to yourself that you will not roll facedown while you are asleep. This is a form of self-hypnosis and seems to program your brain to obey your command unconsciously.

When do my stitches come out?

Usually three to five days after surgery.

How much "down time" will I need?

Because your eyelids will be swollen, you should not drive for about five days, or at least until your stitches come out. In rare instances, the eyes swell shut temporarily, but this is no cause for alarm. After seven days, you can wear a brush-on makeup—but not eyeliner, which should not be applied for at least two weeks. If you do not want anyone to know you had eyelid surgery, you should wait ten to fourteen days before going out in public. That is how long it usually takes for the bruises to fade. Some patients go out sooner but wear dark sunglasses to hide their black-and-blue marks.

Joan, the consultant, did not suffer postoperative pain and healed within a week. "I had minimal black-and-blue marks and no yellowing. I was able to go out in just two days," Joan says. "I had expected much worse." Her only symptom was some transient itchiness. Joan credits her rapid recovery to nature and to carefully following her surgeon's instructions to ice her eyes continuously during her recovery period.

How much followup care should I expect from my surgeon?

Your surgeon will want to see you twenty-four to forty-eight hours after surgery to make sure there is no bleeding or infection. You will return three to five days after surgery to have your stitches taken out. Followup visits are usually scheduled for two weeks later, a month later, three months, and six months later.

How long will it take until the full effects of the surgery are evident?

Usually in ten days, and certainly by two weeks. Scars will remain red for four to six weeks before they fade enough to be virtually undetectable. Scars on African-Americans tend to grow darker than surrounding skin. Most women have no trouble covering their scars with makeup.

Will the shape of my eyes look different after surgery?

Probably, but the change will be subtle. Most patients find an eyelid-lift leaves their eyes looking wider and more open. Joan's large brown eyes were oval before surgery. Now they are round. The change was somewhat surprising to her. "In retrospect, I probably would have asked my doctor to preserve the shape of my eyes," Joan says. "This is something I never thought of before surgery."

Will my eyes be symmetrical after the surgery?

No two eyes are perfectly symmetrical to begin with, and if you are extremely critical, you will certainly see differences in your eyes after surgery. However, a good surgeon strives to make the eyes as symmetrical as possible; indeed some eyelid surgeries are done primarily to make asymmetrical eyes more alike.

What are the chances that I'll need touchup surgery after my blepharoplasty?

About 5 percent of patients need a touchup to further improve the surgical results. This can sometimes be planned before the first operation. One problem necessitating a touchup is the presence of secondary bags, or "festoons," just below the primary bags. The laser peel (see Chapter Seven) is currently in vogue as a way to correct secondary bags, which consist of puffy, sagging skin and a little fat.

It is important that the surgeon remove slightly less lower lid skin than he or she thinks is necessary during the primary eyelid-lift. That lessens the chance of an ectropion occurring. If the surgeon takes off too much skin during the original blepharoplasty, surgically correcting the problem later becomes difficult.

What is the expected life span of the blepharoplasty?

It is difficult to predict the longevity of the eyelid-lift, but it should last about five to ten years or longer.

Can I safely repeat the procedure?

Blepharoplasty of the upper lids can be repeated if necessary. If the lower lids start to sag after a number of years, you probably need a canthopexy ("belt-tightening" procedure) since the skin below has probably been lifted as much as possible.

How much does blepharoplasty cost?

Surgeons' fees for upper and lower blepharoplasty on both eyes range from $2,000 to $5,000. That fee should include a year's worth of followup care. Anesthesiology services cost another $300 to $1,200, depending on the type of anesthesia used and who administers it—a nurse anesthetist or anesthesiologist. Additionally, patients are charged $750 to $2,000 for use of the surgical facility. Office-based operating rooms are at the lower end of that scale; hospital-based facilities are at the upper end.

I hate putting on eyeliner. Is cosmetic tattooing a practical alternative?

If convenience is your sole motivation, cosmetic tattooing—also known as permanent makeup and "micropigmentation"—is probably too risky a solution. You could suffer an infection, eyelash loss, ectropion (basset-hound lids), or injury to the eyeball. In fact, many surgeons are hesitant to tattoo eyelids unless the woman has Parkinson's disease, poor hand-eye coordination, or severe visual impairment that prevents her from applying her own makeup.

Aside from the medical risks, there are social risks associated with any form of permanent cosmetics. Fashions change as do people's color preferences. Permanent eyeliner is forever, as are permanent eyebrows, lipstick, and cheek color. Would you want to wear the same color lipstick and rouge for the rest of your life?

What happens during the procedure?

Using a hand-held device, the physician injects the pigment underneath the skin with a series of thin needles that puncture the skin hundreds of times per minute.

How long does the procedure take?

Thirty to sixty minutes, in most cases.

Will the tattoos hurt afterward?

No. You may develop a little crusting of the eyelid skin for several days. To prevent infection, the lids must be cleansed and coated with a prescription antibiotic ointment until the skin heals.

Does permanent eyeliner fade over time?

After a couple of years, the tattoos will turn lighter and the lines will become less sharp. Sun exposure hastens that effect. At that time, you may desire a touchup.

Who applies permanent makeup?

These procedures can be done by a plastic surgeon, ophthalmologist, or tattoo artist. Be extremely wary of paraprofessionals—such as unlicensed tattoo artists—who offer permanent eyeliner in particular. Unlike physicians, paraprofessionals may not be appropriately trained in proper sterilization techniques. Only licensed physicians can legally administer a local anesthetic. Tattoo needles are painful. Blinking and jerking your head around in pain as needles are injecting dye millimeters from your eyeball is a potential disaster in the making. At the very least, you should wear steel contact lenses during the procedure to protect your eyes. You should also have a "scratch test" before the procedure to make sure you are not allergic to the tattoo pigment, which contains organic compounds and iron oxide. The sterile pigments that physicians use cost more than the average tattoo artist will spend. Tattoo artists usually use nonsterile "bulk" pigments that can be purchased at a fraction of the cost.

How much does micropigmentation cost?

Costs range from several hundred dollars to about $2,000, depending on the type of cosmetic tattoo.

❖ 4 ❖

ABOUT FACE

Face-Lifts

How long have people been getting face-lifts?

The face-lift was born around the turn of the century. Early operations included little more than snipping away a bit of skin in front of the ears. With each subsequent decade, surgeons became bolder and bolder. More aggressive face-lifts achieved better results but were riskier to patients' health. Today, there are a half-dozen major types of face-lifts, each of which has numerous variations to suit individual needs. Complication rates have shrunk markedly in recent years, but a face-lift is still considered major surgery.

What is the goal of a face-lift?

The goal of the face-lift, or rhytidectomy, is to rejuvenate your appearance by reversing some of the ravages of age. To achieve this goal, excess skin and fat are removed from the neck and lower half of the face, and the remaining tissue is tightened. Additionally, vertical bands in the neck are removed, the jowls are reduced to give a smooth border to the jaw, and the folds of skin between the cheeks and lips are lessened.

Until the last year or two, all face-lifts were, in actuality, neck-lifts because they focused on tightening neck skin, and reducing jowls, double chins, and the two prominent bands

69

of muscle that contribute to "turkey-gobbler neck." The primary goal of the newest face-lifting technique, the central face-lift, is to flatten out nasolabial folds—those deep creases between the nostrils and the corners of the mouth. The central face-lift also raises "malar pads" in the cheeks. In young people, these pads of fat accentuate the cheekbones, but they often slip downward as a person ages.

How old is the typical face-lift patient?

Most are in their late forties, although face-lifts are also sought by people in their fifties, sixties, and seventies. The central face-lift is generally geared for people in their forties who have deep nasolabial folds but do not yet have jowls or redundant neck skin. Both traditional and central lifts can be done in one operation.

Is there a way to tell how I might look after a face-lift?

Lie on your back and hold a mirror in front of your face. That image is what you might reasonably expect to achieve with a face-lift. Pulling your skin back with your fingers distorts your face and is an unreliable way to predict what you might look like.

How many face-lifts are performed annually in the United States?

In 1994, the most recent year for which data are available, there were anywhere from 32,283 to 55,400 face-lifts performed in this country.

Are most people satisfied with their face-lifts?

Yes, as long as their expectations were realistic prior to surgery. Satisfied patients understood before surgery that they will never look twenty again. They expected to still look their age after surgery—but better for their age.

What are the most common reasons people are disappointed after their face-lifts?

People who anticipated seeing beauty where there was no beauty before are bound to be disappointed. Others are displeased because every last wrinkle was not removed. Still others mistakenly expected their face-lift to change their bone structure or facial proportions. If you never had high cheekbones and a good jaw line, you will not have them afterward.

What are the limitations of the face-lift?

A face-lift corrects big sags, not fine lines and small wrinkles. It does not erase crow's feet or lines radiating from the lips. The operation does not affect the eyes, brow, or forehead. Traditional face-lifts have less of an impact on nasolabial folds than patients and their surgeons would like. The central face-lift is very limited to the central face region and does not improve jowls, sagging neck skin, or double chins.

Face-lifts do nothing for skin quality or texture. A face-lift cannot, for example, shrink pores or restore a youthful glow to dry, weather-worn skin. To improve skin quality, you can have a chemical peel or dermabrasion (see Chapter Six), or laser peel (see Chapter Seven), which evens out skin tone, tightens skin, and is the only treatment that reduces pore size. Although many people combine their face-lifts with a laser peel, chemical peel, or dermabrasion, these fine-wrinkle-reducing procedures can only be performed on areas that have not been lifted, such as around the mouth.

What distinguishes one face-lift technique from another?

In general, face-lifts are distinguished by how deeply the surgeon cuts. The most superficial lift cuts only the skin layers—the epidermis and dermis. This approach effectively tightens loose skin but is seldom used (though it is regaining popularity) because if jowls are present, the required pull on the skin could distort the mouth.

A more natural look is achieved with the two-layer face-lift, which has been the most popular type of face-lift in the United States since the early 1980s. The surgeon separates the skin from its underlying layer of fibrous fatty tissue and lifts both layers independently of one another. The underlying tissue controls the sagging jowls, thereby allowing the surgeon to pull the skin with less tension. This lessens the chance of stretching out the lips and also decreases the chance of scarring caused by pulling too hard on the skin.

Next come the deeper face-lifts: The "composite face-lift," where the skin and fibrous/fatty layer are lifted as one unit; and a variety of deeper techniques, in which soft facial tissue and skin are dissected apart and lifted separately. The composite lift has the advantage of improved blood supply to the skin because the attached underlying layers "feed" the skin.

The deeper face-lifts take longer because the surgeon must dissect the layers of tissue, carefully cutting around the nerves and muscles.

The deepest face-lift—the "subperiosteal lift"—cuts clear to the bone. This technique is more useful for correcting the nasolabial folds, but if the jowls and excess neck skin are the problem, a face-lift may also be necessary.

There are some theoretical advantages of the more aggressive lifts, but to date, no one has shown them to be better or more long-lasting than the traditional two-layer face-lift. Indeed, a study published in 1995 had surgeons perform a deep-plane lift on one side of the face and a two-layer lift on the other, and you couldn't tell the difference.

The newest face-lift approach is the endoscopic face-lift, where the surgeon lifts all the soft tissues of the face from the level of the bone using an endoscope placed through small incisions in the hairline (see Chapter One). Since the endoscopic face-lift does not remove skin, it is a very controversial, difficult procedure being performed by only a handful of surgeons.

Which of the face-lifts is the riskiest?

The composite and deep-plane lifts are most dangerous in terms of potential damage to nerves.

How will I be readied for surgery?

Prior to surgery, some laboratory testing is usually necessary. A blood count, a urinalysis, an AIDS test, an electrocardiogram (EKG), and a chest x-ray are typically done. An anesthesiologist will examine you and ask questions about any drug allergies or medical conditions that might affect surgery.

Shortly before surgery, a member of the surgical team will shampoo your hair with antibacterial soap. While you are sitting, the surgeon will mark with ink the fat distribution in the face and neck and other facial landmarks to use as a guide during the operation. You will wear a hospital gown and have sticky pads for the EKG placed on your chest. A blood-pressure cuff will be placed on your arm to help monitor your vital signs during surgery. An antiseptic solution will be applied to your face. You will be either put to sleep with general anesthesia, or you will be sedated with drugs given through an intravenous line in your arm before your face is injected with local anesthesia.

Are incisions made in different places to accommodate the different face-lift methods?

Not usually. The standard lift incision starts in the hairline one to two inches above the ear. The incision descends around the front of the ear, behind the cartilage called the tragus, continues around under the ear, hugs the back of the ear, and ends in the hairline just behind the ear. If fat is to be removed from under the chin, or if the bands of the neck are to be corrected, an additional incision is placed in the natural crease under the chin to provide access.

What happens after the face-lift incision is made?

The surgeon completely frees up the skin (and underlying layers, if necessary) from ear to ear, stretching under the chin and to the nasolabial folds. Excess skin and tissue are trimmed from the cheeks and scalp, and the remaining skin and tissue are sewn into their new positions. Sutures are used to close the incisions around the ears; surgical staples usually close the wounds in the hairline.

The two-layer lift, as well as the skin-only lift, are typically combined with liposuction to remove a double chin (see Chapter Thirteen), and surgical repair of neck muscles. The neck-muscle repair (platysmaplasty) involves sewing the two ends of the muscles together with sutures, creating one continuous muscle instead of a pair of prominent cords down the neck.

How long do the effects of the traditional face-lifts last?

That depends on several factors, including the patient's age, amount of skin resiliency, and future sun exposure. In general though, a face-lift lasts five to ten years, with the average being seven years.

How is the central face-lift done?

The central face-lift is performed through incisions under the lower eyelashes. The incisions, which cut to the bone, are placed in natural skin creases so scars will be difficult to see and easily masked by eye shadow. The surgeon then "undermines" the tissue (lifts it away from the bone) and separates the skin from its underlying fat and connective-tissue layers. The surgeon then suspends the lower layers of tissue with permanent stitches and pulls the cheek skin upward and outward. Excess skin is trimmed away at the incision point before the wound is sewn closed. A canthopexy (lid-tightening procedure) is also done so the lower lid will not be dragged down by skin tension introduced by the primary operation.

How long will the central face-lift last?

Because the procedure is so new, there is no documentation of its longevity. However, the central face-lift is now fully described in the medical literature and shows great promise. Many plastic surgeons are likely to start performing it in the near future.

What risks are associated with the central face-lift?

The biggest risk is a pull down of the lower eyelids, which is why proper tightening of the lids is essential. Patients also risk damage to the nerve that transmits sensation from the cheek, upper lip, and nose. This nerve comes out of the bone and goes into the mass of tissue being undermined and lifted during the operation. The surgeon must take great care not to cut or injure this nerve.

Can I have a face-lift as an outpatient?

Yes. Every version of the face-lift can be performed in a properly equipped office surgical suite or other ambulatory operating room.

What are my anesthesia options?

There are two: local anesthetic coupled with intravenous sedation, or general anesthesia. Having local anesthesia lessens the risk of nausea and vomiting that are associated with general anesthesia. If you vomit within twenty-four hours after surgery, it can cause bleeding under your facial skin, a major complication that may require a second trip to the operating room. Local anesthesia may be less expensive than general anesthesia, depending on the financial arrangements with your surgeon and the personnel he or she employs. Be warned, however, that anesthesia selection is not a good area of life in which to cut corners. Local anesthesia may, however, be your only option if your doctor's operating suite is not equipped to provide general anesthesia.

The disadvantage to local anesthesia with sedation is that you are conscious during the operation and must lie still for two-and-a-half to five hours while the doctor operates.

How much pain is associated with a face-lift?

With proper sedation and pain-killing medication, the procedure itself should not be uncomfortable. Afterward, the vast majority of patients report surprisingly little pain. The main sensation is numbness. In cases where the neck muscle is altered, there is a sensation of tightness in the neck. Most patients need codeine to get them over the first twenty-four to thirty-six hours after surgery. By then, any residual pain is generally mild enough to be controlled with acetaminophen. Heather says she experienced "absolutely no pain" after her combination face-lift/blepharoplasty. "I never took a Tylenol after my nose job, either," she adds.

How much swelling will I experience?

Cover the mirrors in your house because you will probably look like a pumpkin. There is an enormous amount of swelling that takes place after your face-lift. By the time your stitches come out five to seven days after surgery, much of the swelling will have gone down. By the time the staples are taken out of your hairline two weeks after surgery, you'll be ready to get back into action. If you had a subperiosteal lift involving all skin and tissue to the bone, you'll need an additional week before going out in public.

Unfortunately, there is nothing you can do to reduce swelling; even ice doesn't seem to help. Some surgeons prescribe steroids to minimize swelling, but this is controversial.

What kind of bandages will be on my face after surgery?

There is a lot of variation in how surgeons dress their patients' faces. You will probably come out of surgery wearing a mummy-type dressing with holes for your eyes, nostrils, and mouth. That will be replaced by a lighter dressing the next day. All dressings come off two to seven days after surgery.

What are the possible complications of a face-lift?

One to 2 percent of patients develop an infection, which can be treated with antibiotics. A similar percentage have postoperative bleeding (hematoma) severe enough to require more surgery. Bleeding is characterized by intense pain, abnormal swelling, and perhaps blistering of the skin. The surgeon must undo the incisions, find and stop the bleeding, and sew the skin back into place. If small, localized amounts of blood have pooled under the skin, the surgeon may be able to drain it without reopening the incision. Small hematomas are usually harmless and may be allowed to resolve on their own. For reasons not entirely clear, men are more susceptible than women to hematomas after a face-lift.

Another potentially serious complication is skin loss, or necrosis, which occurs when skin cells die because they were robbed of their blood supply. The skin is separated from up to 80 percent of its blood supply during the face-lift. Pulling the skin tight further reduces the amount of blood reaching skin cells. Blood flow to facial skin bounces back to much higher levels ten days to three weeks following surgery, but the blood supply never goes back to normal.

The risk of skin loss is twenty times higher in smokers than nonsmokers. That is why many plastic surgeons refuse to do face-lifts on smokers, opting instead for laser peels (see Chapter Seven), liposuction (see Chapter Thirteen), and other less invasive procedures. Nonsmokers must stay away from secondhand smoke for at least a week after a face-lift, when their skin is more vulnerable to necrosis. Symptoms of skin loss begins with blistering that progresses to a purplish blotch. The surgeon may try to salvage dying skin with an antibiotic cream. The most common cases of skin necrosis occur behind the ear and are usually no larger than a dime. A worst-case scenario affects the full thickness of the skin in a region that cannot be covered by hair. There have been cases where half a cheek has been lost to skin necrosis.

Another potential problem is injury to the nerve that controls the facial muscles, in particular the muscles that elevate the eyebrow, close the eye, and control the smile. If smile muscles are injured, the patient can look like she suffered a stroke. Permanent nerve damage is very rare, although it is not uncommon to have a temporary injury to facial nerves as a result of swelling. Temporary nerve damage usually resolves itself in two to three weeks, when swelling subsides. If muscle function does not return in three months, nerve damage is more likely to be permanent and may require additional surgery. The risk of nerve damage associated with the traditional two-layer lift is about 1 to 2 percent. With deep-plane and subperiosteal face-lifts, the risk of nerve damage can be 5 percent or higher.

What can I do to reduce my risk for complications?

Not smoking is the most important step you can take. If you are a smoker and can find a surgeon willing to perform your face-lift, you must shun cigarettes for a minimum of two weeks before and after surgery.

Controlling high blood pressure is also crucial. Hypertension is the leading cause of hematoma in face-lift patients. If you have high blood pressure, your surgeon should not operate unless your pressure is extremely well-controlled by medication.

For up to three weeks after surgery, avoid taking any

drugs that may cause nausea and vomiting. You must also refrain from vigorous exercise, bending at the waist, and sleeping on your face during the same three weeks. Do not fly until two weeks after a face-lift because changes in air pressure might trigger bleeding.

Aside from hypertension, are there other medical conditions that would make me a poor candidate for a face-lift?

Diabetes, vascular diseases, and connective-tissue disorders, such as rheumatoid arthritis, scleroderma, and lupus all diminish the blood supply to the skin, which interferes with proper healing.

The best face-lift candidate has a good overall health status. Some plastic surgeons insist that patients over age fifty get clearance by their internist before undergoing surgery. Anyone over age sixty would be well served by having an exercise stress test prior to surgery to rule out heart disease.

How much scarring will I have?

All face-lift techniques are designed so tension-bearing scars are hidden behind the ear and in the scalp. Wherever there is tension, there is a wide scar. Only a hairline scar should be visible in front of the ear, although this scar is sometimes wider than the patient would like. Women can hide the scar with hair and makeup. Hiding scars is more problematic for men, especially if they have receding hairlines.

How much younger will I look after a face-lift?

That varies from person to person. Now that her sagging skin and jowls are gone and her cheeks and eyelids are tighter, Heather estimates she looks eight to ten years younger—like she did when she was in her late forties. Her result is fairly typical among face-lift patients.

Will I lose any hair?

In most cases, hair loss occurs only along the scar, although more extensive hair loss is possible.

What do face-lifts cost?

There is a broad range of face-lift fees, from about $4,000 to $12,000, with some surgeons charging as much as $18,000. The physician's qualifications, reputation, and location all help determine the fee, as does the type of face-lift performed. As a general rule, the deeper lifts are more expensive than the two-layer and skin-only lifts. Your surgeon's fee should also cover a year's worth of followup visits. Expect to pay another $2,000 to $3,000 for anesthesiology and operating room expenses.

How long should I wait before washing my face and hair after surgery?

Your surgeon or nurse will probably wash your hair after surgery. You can shower two days later, washing your hair with a mild baby shampoo that has no dyes or perfumes. Use a mild soap such as Neutrogena, Dove, or Ivory on your face, cleaning your incision areas carefully with your fingertips. Clotted blood should be dissolved with hydrogen peroxide on cotton swabs. After washing your face, coat the incisions with an over-the-counter antibiotic ointment. Continue this routine until all your stitches and staples come out.

When can I wear makeup again?

In about two weeks, after all your stitches and staples are removed.

Should I avoid exercising after a face-lift?

Absolutely do not exercise for about three weeks after surgery because it elevates your blood pressure, which can cause bleeding under the facial skin. For similar reasons, avoid sexual activity for one to three weeks. After three weeks, you can take mild walks and do gentle exercises; just use common sense. You can resume full activities after six weeks.

Is there anything I can do to help my scars fade?

Nature and time are the greatest healers, although massaging your scars beginning three weeks after surgery can speed up their natural resolution. Rubbing Vitamin E oil into your scars won't hurt, but there is no proof it will help, either. The body generally makes a lot of scar tissue in the first three months. Over the next nine months, the scars should settle down and become less apparent. Using sun block on your face is critical during the six months following your surgery; unfiltered sun exposure will color your scars darker than surrounding skin.

How long until the full effects of my face-lift are apparent?

By two weeks, you will appreciate the changes from your lift, but it takes up to three months to realize the full effects. There may be continued fading of scar tissue for up to a year.

Is there a skin-care routine that can enhance or prolong my results?

Limiting your sun exposure and not smoking will maximize the longevity of your face-lift. Skin creams containing Retin-A or glycolic acid can help even out your skin tone, decrease periodic acne, and lessen fine wrinkling.

How many followup visits will I need with my surgeon?

Your surgeon will want to examine your face twenty-four to forty-eight hours after surgery. You will return five to seven days after surgery to get your first set of stitches out. Two weeks after surgery, the staples are removed from your scalp. You probably will have more followup exams after two weeks, a month, three months, and six months. If there are any complications, you will be seen by your surgeon more frequently.

Will my face look natural after a face-lift?

Some face-lifts look natural; others do not. There is a tremendous amount of art involved in performing a face-lift, and there is great variability in the results. A surgeon can perform a flawless, textbook operation, and the patient's face can still look overdone. A simple skin lift, in the hands of a skilled surgeon, can turn out to be perfectly acceptable, whereas a less experienced surgeon would need to perform a subperiosteal lift to create the same look. Wide variations among surgeons, surgical techniques, and individual patients make predicting the outcome of your face-lift, or any cosmetic surgery, virtually impossible.

Can I safely repeat a face-lift?

Yes. Some people have as many as three face-lifts over the course of their adult life. In some ways, a repeat face-lift is easier because the lines of dissection have already been made, and there is usually less bleeding. On the other hand, previous scar tissue can make the surgery more difficult. There is a higher chance of nerve damage in repeat lifts because scar tissue may have altered normal anatomy.

Will my face feel tight after the lift?

Yes. So will your neck. Tightness continues for three or four weeks, when your skin stretches enough to feel normal again.

How obvious will it be to others that I've had a face-lift?

If someone sees your "before" and "after" photographs, they will probably figure it out. Otherwise, except for your extremely observant friends and acquaintances, most people will think you lost weight, changed your hairdo, or just returned from a relaxing vacation.

✤ 5 ✤

JUST CHEEKY

Cheek and Chin Implants

What is the purpose of cheek implants?

Cheek implants create more prominent cheekbones, or "malar bones." Prominent cheekbones are considered aesthetically pleasing in western cultures. Most patients who want cheek implants never had prominent cheekbones and are seeking malar implants to achieve better facial balance.

Another type of cheek implant, the "submalar implant," is designed to rejuvenate an older face whose natural fat pads have sunk below the cheekbones, producing a hollow, aged appearance. Submalar implants are positioned just below the cheekbones to plump up the hollows in the cheeks and produce a mild, lifting effect. Submalar implants are sometimes added during a face-lift or other facial rejuvenation procedure.

How common is cheek-implant surgery?

Not very. According to the latest data from the American Society of Plastic and Reconstructive Surgeons, cheek implants accounted for a mere 0.3 percent of all cosmetic procedures performed in 1994. Chin augmentation is much more common, accounting for about 1 percent of cosmetic procedures overall.

Manhattan Eye, Ear, and Throat Hospital, one of the

highest volume cosmetic surgery hospitals in the country, reported doing only sixty-four cheek implants over a recent eight-year period.

Which anesthesia is used during facial implant surgery?

Cheek implant surgery usually calls for local anesthesia coupled with sedation or general anesthesia. Chin implant surgery can be performed under straight local anesthesia, but only if the patient is quite stoic.

What are cheek and chin implants made of?

Both types of implants are made of a solid but flexible silicone rubber or the newer Gore-tex. They come in a variety of sizes and designs to accommodate a variety of patients.

Is it possible to be allergic to or reject the implant material?

Silicone is perhaps the most inert material that can be implanted in the human body. Of tens of thousands of patients who have received silicone cheek and chin implants, and of millions of people with other pieces of silicone in their bodies, there has been maybe one allergic reaction reported in the medical literature.

How is the size of my cheek implants determined?

Your plastic surgeon will carefully examine and measure your facial features before selecting an implant size that is appropriate for your bone structure. The implant's length is important, as is its thickness, which translates into how much the cheekbone will project off the face. Most plastic surgeons believe cheek implants should be very subtle; big implants look obvious and bizarre.

Can the implants be taken out if they turn out to be too big or too small?

Yes. If the implant size is selected with appropriate care, however, removal should not be necessary. If the implants become displaced, repositioning is possible but may be a challenge to your surgeon.

Where are the incisions made?

There are three methods of placing cheek implants. The most popular incision is inside the mouth between the cheek skin and teeth. This half-inch-long opening, situated in the pocket above the upper molars, leaves no visible scar.

The second incision option is through the lower eyelid, either through the skin, which leaves a scar in the lid crease, or through the underside of the lid, which leaves no visible scar.

If the cheek implants are to be placed during a face-lift (see Chapter Four), they can be positioned through the normal face-lift incisions.

What happens after the incision is made?

The skin and its underlying tissue are raised off the cheekbone, and the implant is placed directly on the cheekbone. The implant can be placed either above or below the periosteum, the thin layer of tissue covering the bone. If the implant is placed above the periosteum, it is usually sutured in place before the incision is sewn closed. If the implant is placed under the periosteum, it does not need sutures because the membrane snaps back, holding the implant in place. Scar tissue that forms over the next three weeks serves to solidly lock the implants in place.

Submalar implants are placed just under the cheekbones to plump up hollow cheeks.

How much pain is involved in cheek-implant surgery?

The actual procedure is not too uncomfortable, as long as appropriate anesthesia and sedation are used. After surgery, patients report remarkably little pain.

How long does the procedure take?

Cheek-implant surgery generally lasts two hours—one hour per cheek.

What risks are associated with cheek implants?

As with any surgery, there is a small risk of infection and bleeding. If the implantation site becomes infected, the surgeon may be forced to remove the implants. Possible sources of infection include untreated gum disease, a loose tooth, and a significant dental cavity, all of which can harbor bacteria near the incision areas.

Another risk of surgery is injuring the nerve that supplies sensation to the eyelid, cheek, nose, and lip skin. Nerves that control the smile muscles can also be injured, as was the case of one twenty-year-old woman whose smile was asymmetrical for a month after her cheek-implant surgery. Fortunately, nerve damage is both uncommon and temporary; it is usually due to swelling around the nerves.

Another possible complication is implant asymmetry. Your plastic surgeon must be extremely careful to place the implants in the exact same position in each cheek. Even a small deviation will be visible and necessitate a followup procedure to correct the problem.

How much swelling and bruising should I anticipate?

Bruising after this procedure is minor because the implants are placed at a very deep level; no muscles are cut. There will be some swelling, but not enough to keep you inside for more than a week after surgery. Your stitches will be taken out in about seven days unless they are dissolvable stitches placed inside the mouth.

What can I do to promote healing and reduce my risk of complications?

Keeping your head elevated lessens the possibility of bleeding in the first few days after surgery. When you lie down, use two pillows under your head. Consume only beverages and soft foods for the first couple of days. When brushing your teeth during the first two weeks after surgery, avoid the areas inside the mouth where the incisions were made. If you sweep your toothbrush across an incision site, you might rip out your stitches. Another way to reduce your infection risk is to rinse with a solution of half peroxide and half mouthwash after eating until your stitches are removed.

Your implants can shift relatively easily during the first three weeks after placement. To prevent shifting, do not lie on your face, touch your cheeks other than to gently wash your face, exercise, or play sports of any kind for a minimum of three weeks after your operation. After three weeks, enough scar tissue has grown around the implants to lock them into position. From that point on, it would take a significant whack to move your cheek implants.

How much does cheek-implant surgery cost?

The plastic surgeon's fee is in the $2,500 range. The anesthesiologist charges about $500. You will be charged another $600 to $800 for the operating room. The implants themselves cost about $125 apiece.

Can chin- and cheek-implant surgery be done in outpatient settings?

Yes. These procedures are almost always performed in surgicenters or office-based operating rooms.

What is the goal of chin augmentation?

Chin augmentation, or mentoplasty, is designed to enlarge a chin that is too small. Some people inherit an abnormally small chin. There also are rare cases in which the chin mysteriously stops growing in childhood.

How much does chin augmentation cost?

The plastic surgeon's fee for this thirty- to sixty-minute procedure is in the $2,000 range. Because chin augmentation is a shorter procedure, anesthesiologist and operating-room fees are slightly lower than they are for cheek-implant surgery.

How is size of the chin implant determined?

Your plastic surgeon will look at the bone structure of your face and make an aesthetic judgment of how big an implant you need, or whether an implant will be sufficient to correct your problem. In making that determination, the doctor will also pay attention to your nose. A small chin makes a normal-size nose look big and a big nose look even bigger. Rhinoplasty (see Chapter Nine) is sometimes recommended as an adjunct to mentoplasty so the chin and nose will balance each other out. Also, the chin implant cannot be so big that it threatens to poke through the skin or slip out of position.

What happens during chin-implant surgery?

In most cases, the implant is placed through an incision in the crease under the chin. Another possible incision site is inside the lower lip, which leaves no visible scar. Once the implant is properly positioned, it is sewn into place and the incision is closed.

For patients with severely deficient chins, there is an alternative, albeit more extensive, form of chin augmentation called a "sliding genioplasty." This procedure is appropriate in cases where the degree of chin advancement required exceeds 7 or 8 millimeters. Sliding genioplasty involves cutting the bone and extending it forward with titanium metal plates and screws. The technique is more complex, risky, and expensive than implant surgery, but it lets the surgeon make major shifts in the chin's projection or configuration. The surgeon's fee for sliding genioplasty ranges from $4,000 to $6,000, and the procedure is usually done in a hospital setting.

What is the healing process like after chin-implant surgery?

Your lower jaw may feel a little stiff for a few days. Your stitches will be removed about five days after surgery. Swelling and bruising should be minimal.

What postsurgical precautions should I follow?

Until your stitches come out, stick to a soft diet and talk as little as possible. If your stitches are inside your mouth, rinse with a solution of half peroxide and half mouthwash after eating. Avoid bending down for about a week, and do not lie on your face for three weeks. It takes that long for scar tissue to lock your chin implant in place.

What complications are associated with chin augmentation?

There is a small risk of infection, bleeding, and improper positioning of the implant. Each of these problems occurs in fewer than 5 percent of cases. The nerves that supply sensation to the chin and lower lip may be injured by this procedure, resulting in temporary or permanent numbness of the area.

Are most patients happy after having their chin augmented?

It is very unusual to have an unhappy patient after chin augmentation unless the implant is out of position. Should that occur, the implant can usually be repositioned under local anesthesia.

How long do facial implants last?

The solid cheek and chin implants currently in use cannot rupture and therefore should be lifetime items. The need to remove them surgically would probably be very unusual.

LOOK MORE A-PEELING

Chemical Peels and Dermabrasion

What is the purpose of a chemical peel?

A chemical peel, or chemosurgery, improves fine lines, multiple wrinkles, skin tone, and irregular pigmentation that are unaffected by a face-lift. The peel works by chemically removing the top layers of skin. This so-called "controlled burn" spurs the growth of new skin, which generally is smoother and more uniform in color than the original skin. The new skin looks younger to the naked eye and under a microscope. The peel can be applied to the whole face or a region of the face, such as the area around the mouth. The neck and backs of the hands can also be chemically peeled, but the best results are achieved on facial skin.

How long have chemical peels been available?

Chemical skin peeling came into vogue in the early 1960s when Thomas Baker, M.D., and Howard Gordon, M.D., Miami plastic surgeons, first reported its potential. The genesis of their technique arose from the observation that people who suffered superficial facial burns often healed with fewer wrinkles than they had before. That observation sprung to mind when they learned that laywomen at some beauty salons had used chemicals to rejuvenate clients' wrinkled skin. Their results were often acceptable, but there was a high incidence of complications. Drs. Baker and Gordon refined their skin-peeling agents and techniques, and their early experiments yielded spectacular results. Nonetheless, the plastic-surgery community was reluctant to believe that deep peels using phenol really worked. As a result, chemical peeling as a medical treatment for skin aging didn't catch on for several years.

By the 1980s, a second, less-invasive peeling agent—trichloracetic acid (TCA)—was introduced. A third category of peels—the "ultralight" or "lunch-time" peel using glycolic acid (one of the alpha-hydroxy acids, or "fruit acids")—was popularized in the early '90s.

How many chemical peels are done annually in the United States?

According to the American Society of Plastic and Reconstructive Surgeons (ASPRS), its member plastic surgeons performed 29,072 peels in 1994, the latest year for which data are available. That statistic excludes peels performed by dermatologists and other nonplastic surgeons. According to the ASPRS, in some regions of the country chemical peeling is among the top five aesthetic procedures in terms of popularity.

What is the biggest difference between the phenol, TCA and alpha-hydroxy acid peels?

The major difference is how deeply they penetrate—and thus how profoundly they affect—skin. The most dramatic improvement is achieved with the most powerful chemical, phenol. Phenol, or carbolic acid, is the active ingredient in Lysol, the cleanser, and Chloraseptic, the sore-throat remedy. In its standard skin-peeling concentration of about 50 percent, phenol penetrates and removes the entire epidermis (outermost skin layers) down to the middle of the dermis, the skin's inner layers. TCA, by contrast, burns off the entire epidermis and only the most superficial portion of the dermis. Glycolic acid, the mildest of the three peeling agents, removes only the outer layers of the epidermis.

How do I know which peel depth is right for me?

That depends on the condition of your skin. If you have pale, lifeless skin and periodic acne breakouts but not too many wrinkles yet, your best bet is the ultralight glycolic-acid peel. Glycolic acid adds life to the skin, improves its color, and decreases acne breakouts. It is typically sought by women in their twenties, thirties, and forties.

If you are in your thirties, forties, or fifties, and your main problem is early wrinkles, brown blotches, or uneven skin tone, you probably would benefit most from a TCA peel.

The deep phenol peel is geared for people in their forties, fifties, or sixties who have sun-damaged skin characterized by numerous fine lines, wrinkles, and uneven pigmentation. The phenol peel is quickly being replaced by the laser peel (see Chapter Seven) since lasers achieve similar results with fewer risks and side effects. Phenol peels will continue to be available to those who cannot afford laser treatments or people who lack access to a surgeon trained in laser peeling.

Who performs chemical peels?

Phenol peels are traditionally done by plastic surgeons; TCA and glycolic-acid peels are done by both plastic surgeons and dermatologists. In some cases, nurses supervised by doctors administer ultralight peels.

How much do chemical peels cost?

A full-face phenol peel ranges from $1,000 and $2,500, a one-time expense. A TCA peel costs $500 to $1,200 per treatment, which is usually repeated every one to two years. Glycolic-acid peels range from $200 to $400 per treatment. Most people need a series of six glycolic-acid peels spread out over several months. The doctor's fee should include routine followup visits.

Isn't putting chemicals on the skin dangerous?

In an uncontrolled setting with a lay person or inadequately trained doctor or inexperienced nurse, the answer is potentially yes. There have been cases, for example, where acid has been splashed into the eyes producing blindness. Poor technique can also result in disfiguring scars. In the right hands, chemical peels pose little danger, and complication rates are extremely low.

Does cigarette smoking reduce the effectiveness of chemical peels?

Overall, nonsmokers tend to heal faster and enjoy better post-peel results than smokers.

Where are chemical peels done?

All glycolic-acid peels and virtually all TCA peels are done in a doctor's office, usually in an examining room. Phenol peels should be done in an operating room in a hospital, doctor's office, or surgicenter. This requirement adds at least several hundred dollars to the cost of a phenol peel, but the increased safety measures in a surgical facility make this a sound investment.

What risk factors are associated with chemical peels?

Doctors have reported a number of cases of injury with all peeling agents. Splashing the chemical in the eyes can result in vision impairment or even blindness. Scarring, while infrequent with TCA and glycolic-acid peels, is relatively more common with deep phenol peels. The same goes for infections and herpes breakouts. Other possible side effects include decreased pigmentation and dark spots.

Chemical peeling is as much an art as it is a science. There are no guarantees of a satisfactory outcome, but the more training and experience your doctor has, the lower your risk for complications.

Is it better to have whole-face peels or "spot peels" on problem areas?

Glycolic acid and TCA peels are almost always applied to the entire face so that the skin looks uniform. Phenol peels can be applied to the full face or to a region of the face, such as the forehead or "perioral" area (around the mouth).

What are the advantages and disadvantages of the phenol peel?

Because phenol penetrates deeply, it is very effective in reducing fine lines and shallow wrinkles and significantly diminishing many deeper wrinkles. It also results in a very uniform, albeit, lighter than normal complexion. No anesthetic is needed while the chemical is applied because the phenol numbs the skin as it penetrates. (A 0.3 percent phenol concentration in Chloroseptic numbs the throat.) A phenol peel needs to be done just once. If you take good care of your skin afterward, the improvements can last the rest of your life.

Phenol peels have a number of potential down sides, the most dangerous being irregular heartbeats (arrhythmias). Arrhythmias can occur if your doctor applies the chemical too quickly. Phenol must be applied very slowly—over the course of at least one hour—to prevent high levels from reaching the bloodstream. As a precaution, patients are hooked to a cardiac monitor while the chemical is applied. People with heart or kidney disease are generally ruled out as candidates for phenol peels.

Another disadvantage is down time. Your face will swell and ooze so much after your phenol peel that you'll want to hide for eight to ten days. Expect a reasonable amount of discomfort, usually requiring codeine for three or four days until healing takes hold. On the tenth day after the peel, you can wear makeup—but you'll want to use an industrial-strength foundation such as Dermablend or Physician's Formula. You'll be able to switch to your regular foundation in about a month.

Peeled skin will be deep pink in color for four to twelve weeks before it starts to fade. Fading will continue for several months until your skin is a few shades lighter than it used to be. Lightening occurs because phenol destroys so many of the skin's pigment-producing cells. There is no proof, but in theory, melanin destruction also raises your skin-cancer risk. For that reason, it is imperative that you wear a strong sunscreen (SPF 15 or greater) whenever you are exposed to direct or reflected sunlight. Tanning salons are strictly off-limits. It is unlikely that you will ever be able to develop a dark tan after a phenol peel, anyway.

Because phenol wreaks havoc on pigment-producing cells, most plastic surgeons and dermatologists won't perform a deep peel on anyone with darker-than-olive skin. Darker skinned individuals could end up with uneven pigmentation or an obvious line of demarcation at the bottom of the jaw.

Like the other types of chemical peels, phenol does not remove pitted acne scars, excess fat, sagging skin, or large creases, such as the nasolabial folds or frown lines.

There is a small risk of infection associated with phenol peels. If you have ever been exposed to herpes simplex or shingles, you are likely to get a breakout unless you take the antiviral drug Zovirax or Valtrex for a day before and at least a week after surgery. Herpes outbreaks during or after a peel can result in permanent scarring.

What happens during a phenol peel?

Deep chemical peels are usually done on an outpatient basis, but some patients require an overnight hospital stay. You will probably be sedated during the procedure, so make sure you have someone to drive you home afterward. Your hair will be pulled back, and your face will be thoroughly washed with acetone to remove oils, dirt, and soap residue. You will lie on an operating table. The phenol solution (usually a mixture of 50 percent phenol and a variety of other chemicals, soap, oil, and water) is applied slowly with a long, cotton-tipped swab. The length of the procedure depends on whether you are having a full-face or partial peel. Your skin turns white at first, then bright red. There may be some superficial bleeding. Before you leave, your surgeon will apply some antibiotic ointment or another moisturizer such as Vaseline. Your face may or may not be wrapped in tape, depending on your surgeon's preference.

How long after the chemical is applied will my skin begin to peel?

Immediately. The peeling takes the form of a raw, oozing wound.

How much swelling will I experience?

Quite a bit. Your face will look like a pumpkin for eight to ten days. Only time can reduce the swelling.

What kind of followup care will I need?

If your face is bandaged, you will return to your doctor in a day or two to have the bandages removed. After two or three days, you can begin to gently wash off the dead, peeling skin with a washcloth twice a day. Use a mild soap such as Dove or Neutrogena. Try not to pull on the peeling skin, as that can cause bleeding. You should use a moisturizing ointment until healing is complete. Avoid sunlight for the first two weeks. Your doctor will probably want to see you a week after the peel, and again in a month.

What are the pros and cons of the TCA peel?

The TCA peel's great advantage is leaving patients with much less swelling and skin lightening compared with the phenol peel. By the same token, TCA is less effective than phenol in smoothing out fine lines and wrinkles. TCA treatment can take as little as thirty minutes. By the time you leave the doctor's office, you will have no pain or discomfort. You can go back to work in four or five days, when your face has healed to the point where you look as though you have a bad sunburn.

You will experience considerable burning pain for five to ten minutes after the TCA is applied to your skin. To take the edge off that pain, your doctor will probably prescribe a little Valium and Percocet to be taken a hour or two before treatment. The results of a TCA peel can be difficult to predict.

What happens during a TCA peel?

Your hair will be pulled back and your face thoroughly cleansed. The TCA solution will be applied to your skin with a long, cotton-tipped swab. As the TCA is applied, your skin will take on a white, frosted appearance, but that gradually resolves by the time you go home.

Like phenol, TCA is left on the skin. It sinks to a certain depth, then stops. How deeply it penetrates can vary widely, depending on the solution's strength, the doctor's technique, and how the skin was prepared before treatment. TCA comes in a 10 percent to 70 percent solution with water. Different concentrations can be used on different areas of the face.

The more strokes the physician uses to apply TCA, the deeper the chemical will penetrate. The doctor may deliberately vary the number of strokes to give a stronger treatment to the most wrinkled regions. The treatment takes about thirty minutes. Redness will subside in a few hours.

TCA penetrates more evenly and results in a more uniform appearance if you use Retin-A cream daily for a minimum of two weeks prior to treatment. Among other effects, Retin-A sloughs off the outermost, nonviable skin cells.

How long after the TCA is applied will my skin begin to peel?

TCA produces a "dry peel," which means your skin will begin to flake off three to five days after treatment. You should be able to use makeup in about five days.

What are the ups and downs of glycolic acid peels?

The greatest advantage to glycolic acid is you can have your peel at noon and go back to work at one o'clock, hence the nickname "lunch-time peel." (Most people take the day off anyway.) The reason is that glycolic acid, like all alpha-hydroxy acids, works at the microscopic level to remove (exfoliate) the outermost epidermal cells. There is a slight, temporary stinging sensation when the solution is applied. Your skin may turn slightly pink for a few hours after treatment, but it is otherwise impossible to tell your skin is peeling.

The trade-off is the subtlety of skin improvements. You and your doctor may be the only people to notice a change in your appearance. Your skin will be slightly smoother and fresher but not necessarily younger-looking. Any amelioration of wrinkles can usually be attributed to slight swelling that temporarily plumps up wrinkles.

Another disadvantage is the number of treatments needed. Typically, patients require three to six ultra-light peels at one-month intervals to achieve the optimal result. A touchup peel can be performed when necessary after the initial series—about every six to twelve months.

What happens during a glycolic acid peel?

Your face is carefully washed and your hair pulled back. For your first treatment, your doctor will probably use a relatively weak solution (20 percent glycolic acid to 80 percent water) and leave it on your face for two minutes before neutralizing the acid with a mild basic solution. Each subsequent treatment will use a slightly stronger concentration of glycolic acid and be left on your face a little longer. By

the time you reach your final treatment, you may have
worked up to a 70 percent solution that is left on your skin
for five minutes before being neutralized. The doctor applies a postpeel moisturizer before sending you on your
way.

Can I drive immediately after a glycolic-acid peel?
Driving after an ultralight peel is not a problem.

Are there side effects after any of the chemical peels?
There usually are no significant side effects to the glycolic acid peels. The most common side effect to phenol
and TCA peels is milia—tiny whiteheads caused by
clogged pores. Milia usually clears up on its own, or you
may need to return to your doctor to have them uncapped
with a needle or sterile blade.

**Is there anything I can do to enhance the outcome of
my chemical peel?**
Using an over-the-counter alpha-hydroxy acid (AHA)
skin cream daily can increase your chemical peel's longevity. If you are having a series of glycolic acid peels, be sure
to use an AHA cream daily between peels, as well.

With TCA peels, there is a mandatory pre- and postpeel
regimen including Retin-A, topical steroid cream, and hydroquinones (skin bleach), all of which should be used
daily for at least two weeks before your peel and two weeks
after your skin heals. Retin-A strips away the outermost
epidermal cells, creating a more uniform skin surface for
the peeling agent. Steroid cream calms the skin irritation
caused by the Retin-A. Hydroquinones switch off the pigment-producing cells, which can react wildly to a peel if
they are in an active state. Following this regimen adds
about $100 to the overall cost of your treatment, but it is
extremely important in getting good results.

Regardless of the type of peel you have, applying a
strong sunscreen (SPF 15 or greater) twenty minutes before

going outdoors will protect your new skin from photoaging. Using makeup with a built-in sunscreen also helps. And avoid cigarette smoke, which hastens the new skin's natural aging process.

Used without a chemical peel, how effective are the alpha-hydroxy creams that are sold at drugstores and cosmetic counters?

These products contain a much lower concentration of alpha-hydroxy acid (AHA) than the preparations to which plastic surgeons and dermatologists have access. Nonetheless, over-the-counter AHAs do appear to be useful in improving skin tone and reducing periodic acne breakouts. They are of limited usefulness in reducing wrinkles, however.

There are scores of over-the-counter AHA creams, and it is impossible to compare them because AHA concentrations are not stated on product labels. They do appear to be safe, although their action on skin is not yet fully understood. In all likelihood, AHAs remove the upper layer of skin cells mechanically, much like Retin-A works chemically. AHAs also have a true medicinal effect.

Are there any drugs I should avoid prior to having my skin peeled?

Chemical peels should not be done on anyone who has taken Accutane within the past two years because exposure to that drug retards healing. No other drugs are known to interfere with chemical peels.

Can I have more than one kind of chemical peel?

If you are dissatisfied with the results of your glycolic acid peels, you can step up to a TCA peel. You can also have one type of peeling agent applied to one region of your face and a different agent applied to other areas. An example of this approach would be using phenol around your mouth and TCA on the rest of your face.

Is there anything I can do to promote skin healing after the peel?

If there is a chance you have a deficiency of zinc or Vitamins A or C, you should take nutritional supplements because these nutrients are necessary for adequate wound healing. Avoiding cigarette smoke can also contribute to more rapid healing. Do not use abrasive cleansers on your face until healing is complete.

Does chemical peeling make me more susceptible to sunburn?

Yes, because both TCA and phenol peels in particular reduce the number of pigment-producing cells or change their activity. As mentioned earlier, getting a deep tan is impossible after a phenol peel. You may be able to get some color back to your skin after a TCA peel. Glycolic acid peels do not influence your susceptibility to sunburn or your ability to tan.

Are there any medical problems that would rule me out as a candidate for chemical peels?

Physicians should be hesitant to do a phenol peel on someone with diabetes because the infection rate would be higher. Peels can be done on most other people, as long as they have no serious chronic diseases, such as kidney or heart disease.

Can chemical peels be done on the backs of the hands or other areas of the body?

Chemically peeling nonfacial skin is an area of controversy and potential danger. Deep peels are strictly limited to the face. Low-concentration TCA peels can be safely done on neck skin. Some doctors would consider a TCA peel or glycolic acid peel on the hands. But if scarring or infection were to occur, it could impair your hands' ability to function. Bleaching with hydroquinones is a safer alternative for getting rid of age spots on the backs of the hands.

Why is facial skin more conducive to chemical peels?

Facial skin heals faster and more completely than other areas of the body. For one thing, the blood supply to the face is much better. Also, facial skin is endowed with more sweat glands and hair follicles, from which new skin grows up.

Can I have a chemical peel with a face-lift?

An old plastic surgery axiom says that areas that have been superficially lifted should not be simultaneously peeled. The current feeling among plastic surgeons is that deeper forehead-, face-, and transconjunctival eyelid-lifts can safely be accompanied by TCA peels. However, people who have had superficial lifts should avoid phenol and TCA peels because the combination injures the skin from below and above—a double insult that can lead to skin destruction.

You can safely have a glycolic acid peel after any type of face-lift, but you should wait a few weeks. Lifted skin can be peeled by any technique about a month after surgery.

Are there any circumstances under which health insurance would cover a chemical peel?

There is some evidence that a phenol peel can prevent recurrence of skin cancer in patients who have a history of the disease. If this is your situation, you may be able to persuade your insurer to cover your treatment.

Will my pores be bigger after a chemical peel?

It depends on the type of peel. A phenol peel will probably make your pores larger. Changes in pore size after a TCA peel vary from person to person. Glycolic acid peels often will decrease pore size.

Can I have a peel during an acne breakout?

No. If you are broken out the day your chemical peel is scheduled, postpone the treatment until your face is cleared up. This will decrease your risk of infection.

Will I need to avoid exercise or perspiring after my peel?

Refrain from strenuous physical activity for ten days to two weeks after a phenol peel and for about a week after a TCA peel to give your skin time to heal. Perspiring is not a problem after glycolic acid peels.

How long will it take to see the full effects of my chemical peel?

With the glycolic acid peel, the effects are cumulative; your skin looks slightly better within a week after each peel in the series. You'll see the maximum effect of a TCA peel as soon as your skin heals. It takes one or two months for the effects of your phenol peel to be fully evident.

It is important to realize that swelling, which occurs in different degrees with each type of chemical peel, can make your face appear remarkably wrinkle-free. When the swelling subsides, you may see the reemergence of some wrinkles that you thought were gone.

How do chemical peels differ from dermabrasion?

While peels work chemically to remove skin layers, dermabrasion removes skin mechanically. The doctor operates with a motor-driven, hand-held device called a "dermabrader," which holds a rapidly rotating wire brush or sander. The dermabrader removes the entire epidermis and variable depths of the dermis. Unlike peels, which remove skin to relatively uniform depths, the dermabrader can remove "peaks" and leave "valleys" to flatten out scars. Phenol, TCA, and glycolic acid don't know the difference between scar tissue and normal skin.

What are the goals of dermabrasion?

As alluded to above, dermabrasion's primary use is to smooth out pitted acne scars and isolated raised scars on the face and other body sites, such as the legs and back. It has also been combined with a chemical peel in a procedure known as "chemabrasion" to reduce stubborn wrinkles around the mouth.

How effective is dermabrasion?

In a best-case scenario, dermabrasion reduces acne scars by about 50 percent, but the majority of patients achieve only a 10 percent to 30 percent improvement. Patients must have very realistic expectations going into the procedure and understand that they might need a second dermabrasion. However, people who have endured severe acne scars for years have been happy with even a partial improvement. Dermabrasion is somewhat more successful in flattening out raised scars.

How popular is dermabrasion?

Laser peels (see Chapter Seven) have rendered dermabrasion practically obsolete. Dermabrasion was never tremendously prevalent in the past, accounting for just 1 or 2 percent of all cosmetic-surgery procedures. The reason is its limited usefulness and comparatively high risk of complications. Dermabrasion will remain available to people who cannot afford laser surgery, which is more effective, safer, but far more costly.

How much does dermabrasion cost?

Fees for dermabrasion vary enormously, from $300 to $3,000, depending on the doctor's geographic area and how much skin is treated.

Which specialists perform dermabrasion?

Dermabrasion, an office procedure, is done by both plastic surgeons and dermatologists.

Does dermabrasion hurt?

Your skin will first be anesthetized so you feel nothing during the procedure. Many dermatologists briefly freeze the skin; most plastic surgeons inject the area with a local anesthetic. It is after dermabrasion that the real pain sets in. Most patients require a narcotic for three to five days following dermabrasion.

What happens during the healing process?

Healing from dermabrasion is a very messy affair. Your face will be sore like a scraped knee, continually oozing blister fluid that must be washed away four to ten times a day for the first forty-eight hours. You won't want to go out in public for one to two weeks, after which you can wear makeup. Your skin will remain red for one to three months.

How much swelling will I experience after dermabrasion?

There will be some swelling, but it won't be as profound as the swelling after a phenol peel.

What potential complications might arise from dermabrasion?

Residual scarring is a real possibility, especially when aggressive dermabrasion is done. Dermabrading skin around the eyelids poses a danger to the eyes; there have been cases of eyelids being ripped off by a dermabrader. If an infection sets in and is not properly treated, you could wind up with destruction of the dermis at the infection site, resulting in scarring.

Pigment loss due to dermabrasion is also a risk factor, although it is less common with dermabrasion than with chemical peels or laser procedures. This is why doctors treat either the whole face or large anatomical regions; any pigment differences are less noticeable than they would be if treatment were confined to a small spot. In general, people with darker complexions are more likely than those with lighter skin to see some color changes after dermabrasion.

Can dermabrasion be performed during a face-lift operation?

Yes, but only around the mouth.

How many followup visits will I need after dermabrasion?

You will probably return the next day to have your doctor carefully clean your wounds. You will be examined again a week later and a month after that.

How long until I will see the full effects of this procedure?

One to two months.

❖ 7 ❖

ZAP

Ultrapulsed Laser—The Newest Weapon Against Skin Aging

What is an ultrapulsed laser?

The ultrapulsed laser is a nickname for the pulsed carbon-dioxide (CO_2) laser beam—the latest high-tech weapon in the war against wrinkles. Unlike traditional lasers, which deliver a continuous beam of concentrated light energy, the ultrapulse delivers light in tiny bursts. Each burst is so short in duration that any heat it generates dissipates before the next burst. The skin never gets hot enough to burn. It's the same concept as quickly passing your finger back and forth through a candle flame without getting burned.

Cosmetic surgeons, in particular, embraced this new technology when it was introduced in the mid-1990s. Continuous-wave medical lasers had failed miserably in almost all plastic surgery applications because they charred the skin. Charring produces scarring.

How can an ultrapulsed laser make my face look younger?

A pulsed laser vaporizes the top few layers of skin and tightens underlying collagen tissue. Once new skin grows back, fine lines, wrinkles, irregular pigmentation and other symptoms of skin aging are reduced and, in many cases, eliminated. The face looks smoother, silkier, more uniform, and more radiant. Additionally, scars, including those from acne and chickenpox, become less visible. Most patients are thrilled with the results.

Why is this procedure commonly called "laser resurfacing"?

People who market the technology came up with that term, but laser "resurfacing" is a misnomer. It is the human body that does the "resurfacing" by growing back new skin; the laser is a tool that initiates this natural, biological process. A more accurate description would be "laser peeling," "laser vaporization," or "laser desurfacing."

Where are laser peels performed?

Laser peels are done in an operating room, either freestanding or hospital-based.

Which specialists perform laser peels?

The specialists who seek out advanced training in laser peels are primarily plastic surgeons, dermatologists, otolaryngologists (head and neck surgeons), and ophthalmologists. Unfortunately, rising consumer demand for laser peels has prompted some doctors to offer the procedure despite a lack of adequate training. Consumers must be extraordinarily careful in selecting a doctor to perform a laser peel (see Chapter One).

How much training and experience does a surgeon need to be proficient at laser peeling?

It depends on how much training and experience the doctor has had in other forms of laser surgery. Surgeons who have used lasers extensively for other applications can learn laser peeling in an afternoon. Physicians who have never used lasers before should take a full fourteen-hour training course, observe an experienced surgeon performing laser peels several times, and gain hands-on experience before doing it without supervision. Any doctor performing laser peels should have background training in aesthetic surgery in order to properly apply their new technical skills and knowledge.

What kind of anesthesia is used?

A laser peel can be done under local anesthesia with sedation or under general anesthesia. Most surgeons prefer general anesthesia for a full-face laser peel and local anesthesia for peeling only a region of the face such as the forehead, mouth area, cheeks or around the eyes.

How will I be prepared for my laser peel?

Before entering the operating room, your face is cleaned with acetone to remove oils. Prior to surgery, your face is marked out with a surgical pen to demarcate areas to be laser peeled. Betadine antibiotic solution is used to kill bacteria. Anesthetic drops are put in your eyes followed by protective steel contact lenses. If the skin around your mouth is the only area to be peeled, your eyes can be protected by drapes and the contacts are not needed.

Your hair and body are covered with a layer of dry drapes and a second layer of wet drapes to prevent fire in case the laser beam hits the cloth. Anesthesia is administered. Members of the surgeon team don goggles to protect their eyes before the laser is turned on.

What happens next?

The surgeon methodically moves the laser across the skin, generally beginning at the forehead before moving to the eyelids, cheeks, nose, mouth, and jaw. Skin is treated one small area at a time. Depending on the surgeon's needs at the moment, the laser is continually reprogrammed to deliver the beam in dozens of different energy levels and shapes: a relatively large triangular swath; a small, medium or large hexagon; or a fine line, to name a few. Some machines offer a doughnut-shaped option designed specifically for pitted acne scars. In most cases, three passes are made over the skin; the first vaporizes the top layers of skin, and the subsequent passes shrink the collagen layer and remove wrinkles.

If you are awake during the procedure, you will smell smoke as the skin vaporizes, and you will feel some gentle snapping on your skin as the laser does its work. You will also hear the laser's zapping sound as well as its vacuum tube capturing the vapors.

Mary, a fifty-year-old adult education teacher who had her whole face laser peeled under local anesthesia preceded by doses of Percocet and Valium, likened the feeling to "rubber bands snapping on your face."

"But it was tolerable, and I have a low pain threshold," she continues. "I told my doctor that if I could go through this, I'm sure just about everybody could."

How long does the procedure take?

A full face can be laser peeled in as little as forty-five minutes with state-of-the-art technology, which includes a computerized "scanner." Using slightly older ultrapulse technology without the scanner, the procedure can take up to two hours. Operating under general anesthesia takes less time because the patient is spared the additional fifteen minutes it takes to numb the face. A regional laser peel generally takes fifteen to thirty minutes.

How will I look after a laser peel?

At first, your skin will look extremely red and raw, but it will not bleed. The redness will subside over the next seven to fourteen days as the skin heals. Until that happens, your face will appear wet and shiny, with a blistery ooze the first few days. If you look in the mirror during this early phase of recovery, you may cry. If someone rings your doorbell, you won't want to answer. But if you can wait it out, the results are well worth it.

For several weeks after healing, your face will appear wrinkle-free. Unfortunately, this is a temporary side effect of skin swelling. As soon as the swelling goes down in a few weeks, some wrinkles will inevitably return, but the overall appearance of your face will be much improved. (The swelling effect is one more reason to be extremely wary of any "before" and "after" laser-peel photographs you might see. The second picture may have been taken during that window of time before the swelling subsides.)

Will my face be bandaged after surgery?

That is a matter of preference. Your surgeon will probably offer two options for protecting your skin following a laser peel: The closed technique, where the face is bandaged; and the open technique where no bandages are used. There are advantages and disadvantages to both.

For the closed technique, a specific type of tape, most commonly Flexzan, dresses the areas where skin was laser peeled. Flexzan is a sophisticated biomembrane that keeps in moisture, significantly decreases pain, and speeds up healing time. The tape stays on for seven to ten days, during which it must be kept completely dry. That means taking baths instead of showers and having someone else wash your hair. Flexzan will cost the doctor $20 or so for a full-face wrap.

The open technique involves a fair amount of pain and discomfort until healing is completed in ten days to two weeks. You'll probably need some ibuprofen or codeine the first couple of days. Your skin must be washed four to ten times a day with soap and water. Any crusts that form on your face must be dissolved with a water-and-vinegar solution or hydrogen peroxide with each washing. After each wash, you must coat your face with a moisturizing ointment such as petroleum jelly, Preparation H, or Crisco shortening. The moisturizers are essential to prevent drying of the exposed, underlying dermis. This routine must continue until your skin is completely healed.

How much "down time" will I need before I can be seen in public?

If your face is taped, you will probably need to hide out for a week to ten days until your "mummy wrap" comes off. With the open technique, it will be two weeks before your appearance is "socially acceptable." It will take six weeks to three months for pink skin to fade back to your normal skin tone.

How soon after treatment can I wear makeup?

If your face was wrapped, you can use makeup soon after the tape comes off, when all areas are healed. You'll need to wait ten to fourteen days if no bandages were used.

What advantages does laser peeling have over chemical peeling and dermabrasion?

All three techniques remove the epidermis and variable amounts of dermis, but the laser completes its mission with far greater accuracy, precision, and predictability. Ultra-pulsed lasers can be programmed to vaporize skin to the exact depth the surgeon deems necessary for each area of the face. The laser's pulse rate can be adjusted from about ten to 540 bursts per second. The longer the bursts, and the higher the energy of the pulse, the deeper the vaporization of skin.

The surgeon can further fine-tune depth of vaporization by increasing or decreasing the number of passes the laser beam makes over any given section of skin. The most sophisticated pulsed lasers incorporate robotics, which speed up the procedure and increase its accuracy. The laser peel is bloodless because it cauterizes (heat seals) blood vessels as it vaporizes skin. Because no skin is cut or lifted, there is no risk of bleeding under the skin (hematoma) during or after the peel.

The ultrapulse laser's most unique quality, though, is its ability to tighten skin by heating up the underlying collagen (structural) layer. When exposed to heat, collagen shrinks, much like Saran Wrap shrinks when exposed to heat. If you look at the surface area of skin under a microscope before and after it was laser peeled, you would see less skin. Tighter skin translates into fewer, less pronounced wrinkles.

Clearly, the surgeon doesn't have nearly as much control with the dermabrader or chemical peeling agents. As a result, the laser peel may well supplant both dermabrasion and deep phenol skin peels in the very near future.

What are the disadvantages of laser peels?

The laser peel does not reduce sagging jowls, wrinkled necks, or double chins. Because they have more pigment, Asians, Hispanics, and African-Americans are likely to experience light or dark patches on their skin after a laser peel. The laser peel requires a strict pre- and post-peel skin-care regimen, which, if not adhered to, can reduce the peel's effectiveness.

As with other forms of cosmetic surgery, there is a risk of infection, both bacterial and viral. If you have a history of shingles or herpes, you need to take the antiviral drugs Valtrex or Zovirax before and after your laser peel. If infection were to occur, it could cause scarring. Scarring can also result if the laser vaporizes skin too deeply.

A common complication is the development of an "ectropion," or pulling down of the lower eyelids, in response to collagen tightening. Before surgery, the surgeon must carefully assess the laxity and muscle tone of your lower eyelids. If the lid can be easily pulled out from the eyeball and doesn't snap back rapidly, a canthopexy (eyelid-tightening operation) must be performed immediately before the laser peel (see Chapter Three). Many plastic surgeons are finding they need to do a canthopexy in approximately half their laser-peel patients. If the procedure is not performed when indicated, the lid will pull down, potentially exposing the eyeball to drying, ulceration, and infection. These disastrous complications are in addition to an unattractive appearance. Canthopexy adds about $1,500 to $2,000 to your total tab.

Other complications associated with laser include injury to the eyeball, even blindness, if the laser beam hits the eye. If it hits the teeth, it can cause permanent staining of the enamel.

How much does laser peeling cost?

Surgeons' fees for full-face peels range from about $2,500 to $5,000. The fee for a regional peel is about $1,500 to $2,000. These fees exclude operating room and anesthesiology costs.

Why is laser peeling so expensive?

The price tag on an ultrapulsed laser machine runs from $50,000 to $130,000—enough to buy a house. Renting a laser can exceed $1,500 a day.

Not only is the technology expensive, so is marketing it. Anytime you see a laser story in the news media, you can safely bet it originated from a press release from the laser company's marketing department or from a marketing specialist hired by the surgeon.

Are there any advantages to having a full-face laser peel as opposed to a regional peel?

Aesthetically, not really. If done properly, regional peels follow normal anatomical borders, so if slight differences in pigmentation or texture emerge, your face should still appear normal. If cost is a concern, regional peels have an advantage in that they are considerably less expensive.

What can I do to optimize the results of my laser peel?

Avoid cigarette smoke for a minimum of two weeks before and after surgery. Beginning at least two weeks before your appointment, start using Retin-A cream, a topical steroid cream, and hydroquinones (skin bleach) daily, as directed by your doctor. If you have herpes, take the antiviral drug Valtrex for a day before and a week after your peel to prevent breakouts.

If you have taken Accutane within the last eighteen to twenty-four months, you cannot have a laser peel because the medication interferes with healing by inhibiting the re-growth of new skin.

How much improvement should I expect after a laser peel?

It is reasonable to anticipate a dramatic improvement in static wrinkles, those that are visible when the facial muscles are relaxed. No cosmetic surgery, including laser peels, can eliminate "dynamic" wrinkles, such as smile lines that form when the face is animated without directly removing the causative muscle. Dynamic wrinkles are produced by the buckling of skin over contracting muscles; if you look at a seventeen-year-old's face, you'll see them there, too.

You will have significant shrinkage of facial scars, both pitted and raised, after a laser peel. Overall, the improvements after a laser peel are overwhelmingly more dramatic than those achieved with chemical or mechanical skin peeling.

How long will the improvements last?

No one knows for sure because the technique is too new. Some experts speculate a laser peel's shrinking effect on collagen may be temporary; the shrunken fibers could stretch out over time, causing some wrinkles to reform. Only long-term studies will give surgeons more definitive answers. In theory, though, overall skin improvement should last many years, if not decades. If you want your new skin to stay young looking, you must avoid cigarette smoke and reduce your exposure to ultraviolet light as much as practical. Because UV rays penetrate clouds, you should apply heavy-duty sunscreens to all exposed skin whenever you spend more than a few minutes outside during the day.

Mary has resigned herself to the fact that tanning is no longer part of her life. "I've got to stay out of the sun, and I'll always have to wear sunscreen, like (SPF) 23," she says. "I'll never tan my face, ever. When I see people doing that now, I just cringe."

Will the laser peel replace the face-lift?

Not by itself. The face-lift is still superior when it comes to removing loose, hanging skin, such as the jowls, and tightening underlying muscle tissue. After healing from a face-lift, you can have a laser peel.

In certain individuals, a combination of less-invasive procedures can replace a face-lift. For instance, you can undergo a laser peel to smooth out your skin texture, liposuction to remove excess fat from your jowls and from under your chin, surgery to eliminate muscle bands in your neck, and perhaps some minor alterations of underlying face and neck tissue. This constellation of procedures would cost about the same or more than a face-lift, but you would need fewer incisions and run a lower risk of hematomas and bad scarring. People under age sixty would benefit most from such an approach.

Which cosmetic procedures are most commonly combined with laser peels?

One typical companion procedure is the transconjunctival lower eyelid lift, which uses an incision inside the lower lid. Since there is no cutting on the skin's surface, an ultrapulse laser can finish the job by reducing wrinkles around the eyes.

It is also common to combine laser surgery with an endoscopic brow-lift and facial liposuction of the double-chin and jowls.

Can other parts of the body, such as the hands, be resurfaced by laser?

Laser peels are ineffective in minimizing stretch marks

on the abdomen but have been advertised for this purpose. However, consumers must realize that, as of this writing, there has never been a scientific study showing that the laser is effective on stretch marks. Beware of anecdotes that may be promulgated to help "sell" this expensive technology; the plural of "anecdote" is not "data." It would be awfully risky to attempt laser peeling other body parts, especially the hands. If scarring or infection occurred, it could be functionally devastating.

What kind of followup schedule will I need with my surgeon?

Your surgeon will want to see you one or two days after your peel to remove any accumulations of crusts and to reapply your bandages, if necessary. You will return seven to ten days after surgery to have your bandages removed. The surgeon will want to check you out again about two weeks later, and a couple of months after that.

Can a laser peel be repeated?

Probably, but the technology hasn't been around long enough for someone to need a repeat laser peel of the whole face. The ultrapulse laser has been safely used to touch up residual wrinkles several months after healing from an initial laser peel.

What other cosmetic applications do lasers have?

Various other types of lasers can be used to correct portwine stains, spider veins on the face (see Chapter Seventeen), and to remove brown, pigmented areas and tattoos.

✦ 8 ✦

YOUTH IN A SYRINGE

Filling Wrinkles with Fat and Collagen

What are injectable fillers?

Injectable fillers are substances that are implanted or injected beneath the skin's surface to plump up lines, wrinkles, creases, and depressions, or to make the lips fuller.

What sorts of substances are used?

The filling substances used most often are the patient's own fat, called "autologous fat grafts"; and bovine collagen, a fibrous protein derived from cowhide. Fibrel, a less frequently used filling substance, is derived from pig collagen and must be mixed with the patient's own blood before being injected. A new technique utilizes cadaver skin that has been processed to remove all the cells, leaving behind a human-collagen matrix, or "soft-tissue graft."

Another injectable filler, liquid silicone, was used in the past but is now illegal due to serious safety concerns.

Is there such a thing as a human collagen graft?

Yes. This type of dermal graft has been done for years. An incision is made in the buttocks or groin, and a piece of skin is harvested. The epidermis is removed from the harvested skin and the dermis is shaped. The surgeon then makes a tunneling incision on the wrinkle or depression to

118

be filled in, inserts the graft, and closes the incision. In time, the graft becomes integrated into the surrounding tissue. A very faint, tiny scar is left behind. The donor site scar may be substantial, however. Human collagen from donors is now being marketed. This is entirely different from your own (autologous) collagen.

What are the advantages and disadvantages of human collagen as a skin filler?

Human collagen is less likely than cow collagen to trigger an allergic response. However, there is a theoretical risk of transmitting an infectious disease, such as AIDS or hepatitis, from the donor to the recipient of a human collagen graft.

Of the two most popular filling substances, fat and bovine collagen, which is better?

Both have advantages and disadvantages, but fat grafting is safer and could be expected to last longer than collagen injections.

Which skin irregularities are most responsive to fat grafts?

Fat grafts are most useful for filling in skin depressions, large wrinkles, crags, and deep skin creases, including nasolabial folds. Fat can be grafted to skin on the face and almost anywhere else on the body, except the backs of the hands and the breasts (it is malpractice to inject any filling substance into the breasts). Autologous fat grafts are also used to plump up thin lips. (So-called ''lip augmentation'' can also be achieved with dermis taken from the patient's own skin or with the synthetic material Gore-tex.)

Who is a typical candidate for fat grafting?

Middle-aged patients who want to flatten out their nasolabial folds are the most common group seeking this procedure.

When it comes to lip augmentation, there are two age groups plastic surgeons typically see: Young models and people in their twenties who want to look like a model; and women in their midfifties who wish to restore some bulk to lips that have grown thinner with age.

Where is fat grafting usually performed?

Fat grafting is an outpatient procedure that is performed in an office-based, freestanding, or hospital-based surgical facility.

What happens during the procedure?

You are given an oral analgesic and sedative to make you more relaxed. Antiseptic medication is applied to the donor and graft sites. Lidocaine, a local anesthetic, is injected into the donor site, usually the neck (double-chin area), buttocks, or abdomen. Your surgeon may ask for your input on where you want some fat removed. A small incision, usually less than one-quarter inch, is made at the donor site. The surgeon places a large-gauge needle through the incision and gently vacuums out a few ounces of fat into a syringe. The amount of fat taken depends on how many lines you want filled and how deep they are. The harvested fat is then separated from blood and anesthetic fluid, a task that generally takes less than three minutes.

Up until a couple of years ago, the fat would then simply be injected through a needle into the lips, wrinkle, or depression. Surgeons now realize that injection destroys fat cells. Only living cells are more likely to be incorporated permanently into neighboring tissue. The current protocol, therefore, is to lift up the skin and lay the fat in its new location through a tiny, well-hidden incision, about one-eighth of an inch long. This technique, done under local anesthesia, is designed to keep the fat graft alive and healthy and doesn't squeeze it into tissue under high pressure. Blood vessels soon branch into the transplanted fat tissue, just as blood vessels grow into skin grafts on burn victims.

The incisions at the donor and graft sites are closed with one or two stitches. After a couple hours in the recovery room, you are sent home.

What is the healing process like?

You'll need about two days of down time before the swelling at the graft site subsides. You will experience some black-and-blue marks and numbness at both donor and graft sites for a couple of weeks. Over-the-counter ibuprofen or acetaminophen can usually control any discomfort. If you cover the visible bruises with makeup, you can go about your business immediately after treatment.

How long does fat grafting take?

Anywhere from thirty to ninety minutes, depending on the number of areas being treated.

What are the main advantages to fat grafts?

In many cases, if the procedure is done properly, the improvements should be permanent. The majority of patients need only one graft to achieve their desired results; second fat grafts are required in only 10 to 20 percent of cases. There is zero risk of allergy or rejection because your immune system recognizes the graft as your own tissue.

What are the main disadvantages to fat grafts?

Fat is not terribly effective on small lines and shallow wrinkles. Neither fat nor any other filling material should be implanted or injected near the eyes because it can cause blindness.

Another disadvantage is that patients must endure, and pay for, a two-step procedure—harvesting and grafting. The average surgeon's fee for filling in nasolabial folds and other large creases is about $800, including fat harvesting. Lip augmentation costs closer to $1,500 or $2,000. You will be charged another $300 or more for use of the operating room. Several grafts can be completed in one operation, but the more grafts you have, the more expensive the operation becomes.

Fat-graft patients run a small risk of infection and will have small scars at both the donor and graft sites.

Which defects can be corrected with bovine collagen injections?

Collagen is approved by the U.S. Food and Drug Administration for filling in "contour deformities" in the skin, such as acne scars and wrinkles. It can also be used on nasolabial folds and to fill in fine vertical lines on the skin bordering the mouth. It is not approved for augmentation of the lips or any other area of the body.

Who is a typical candidate for bovine collagen implants?

The average candidate is looking for a quick-fix, albeit temporary, improvement with no down time. These individuals are usually interested in filling in the small lines around their lips or flattening out their nasolabial fold.

What happens during a collagen-injection procedure?

The skin is thoroughly washed and painted with an antibacterial solution. The collagen is injected through a syringe along the length of each wrinkle until a 10 percent overcorrection is achieved. Overcorrection prolongs the treatment's effectiveness because the body eventually "digests" the collagen implants. You will experience some temporary discomfort during the injections, but not enough to warrant local anesthesia. Collagen injections are usually administered in the doctor's examining room.

What are the advantages of bovine collagen?

In liquid form, bovine collagen is readily available in prepared syringes. The procedure is completed in a matter of minutes since no harvesting or preparation is needed. Patients are fully recovered in two or three hours.

Initially, collagen injections are less costly than a fat graft, about $300 per syringe. A single syringe usually has enough collagen to treat multiple scars and wrinkles. However, the necessity for periodic injections to maintain your appearance drives up the overall cost of collagen treatments.

What are the disadvantages of collagen injections?

Some specialists have linked serious health problems to collagen injections. Polymyositis and dermatomyositis are two crippling and often fatal collagen diseases that "seem to be related to (patients') prior collagen injections that took place over a period of time," writes Steven M. Hoefflin, M.D., in the medical text, *Practical Procedures in Aesthetic Plastic Surgery: Tips and Traps* (Springer-Verlag, 1994). There is further suspicion that bovine collagen injections may play a role in the development of autoimmune diseases such as rheumatoid arthritis.

Hoefflin points out that recipients of bovine collagen injections can develop antibodies, which destroy the collagen implant. Antibodies form when the body recognizes something as a foreign substance. Some doctors believe that with progressive injections of bovine collagen, the body makes a higher number of antibodies, which digest the implants at an increasingly faster rate. While bovine collagen has been administered to thousands of patients without incident, some surgeons, including Hoefflin, have suspended their use of collagen implants until more is known about the potential side-effects.

How can I find out if I am allergic to bovine collagen?

Your doctor will inject a small bead of collagen under the skin in your forearm. If the area grows irritated over the next four weeks, you are not a candidate for collagen injections. A small percentage of people whose skin test reveals no immediate allergy will develop a collagen sensitivity over time. According to the Food and Drug Administration, collagen allergies can take the form of "rash, hives, joint and muscle pain, headache, and in a few cases, severe reactions that include shock and difficult breathing." Other adverse effects that appear to be related to collagen injections include infections, abscesses, open sores, lumps, peeling of the skin, scarring, recurrence of herpes simplex, and partial blindness, according to the FDA.

About 3 percent of the population is allergic to bovine collagen and should not receive the treatments. Nor should individuals with severe allergies to numerous other substances, the FDA warns.

How long will a bovine collagen implant stay in my skin?

There is no way to predict how long the treatment will last in any given patient. Most people find they need followup injections in two to six months, although there are documented cases of collagen injections lasting as short as two weeks and as long as two years.

Are there any medical conditions that would make me an unsuitable candidate for collagen injections?

Yes. Collagen should not be injected into anyone with a connective tissue disease such as rheumatoid arthritis or scleroderma. Collagen injections should be done with extreme caution in diabetics.

What's involved in Fibrel injections?

Fibrel is injected in the same manner as bovine collagen, but Fibrel requires considerably more preparation. Blood must be drawn from the patient and placed in a centrifuge before being mixed with the pig collagen. The complexity of administering this material is probably the main reason why Fibrel is the least popular filling substance currently in use.

What does a Fibrel injection cost?

You will be charged about $200 to $600 per injection.

Which specialists correct wrinkles and other skin irregularities with filling substances?

Dermatologists and plastic surgeons are trained to use filling substances, although fat grafting is performed primarily by plastic surgeons.

How do filling substances compare with laser and chemical peels in smoothing out wrinkles and acne scars?

Fillers are probably not as effective as laser and chemical peels for correcting small lines and wrinkles. However, fat grafts are probably superior to the laser for minimizing large skin depressions, creases, and folds.

Can implanted collagen or fat drift around my body?

Such an occurrence is unlikely.

Are injectable fillers appropriate companion treatments to skin peels and face-lifts?

Absolutely. In fact, fat implantation or collagen injections can be done in the same operation as a skin peel with TCA or glycolic acid (see Chapter Six). Be sure your surgeon is properly trained in the latest filling procedures. Your cosmetic surgeon may not necessarily know how to do them.

How deep must the filling substances go to do their job?

That is determined by the depth of skin defect being treated. In general, collagen is injected no deeper than the dermis. Fat is grafted beneath the dermis, in the normal fat layer, to fill deep lines and folds.

Why are silicone injections illegal in the United States?

There are too many potentially adverse side effects, according to the FDA, which has not approved liquid silicone for any cosmetic purpose. Adverse effects may include silicone drift to other parts of the body, inflammation and discoloration of surrounding tissues, and the formation of nodules of granulated, inflamed tissue. If silicone-treated tissue becomes infected, the only treatment may be surgical removal of the skin, a cosmetically devastating procedure.

❖ 9 ❖

NOSE ANEW

Rhinoplasty

Where does the word "rhinoplasty" come from?

"Rhino" is derived from the Latin word for "nose." The rhinoceros is so named because of the giant horn protruding from the middle of its face. "Plasty" means to mold. Informally referred to as "nose jobs," the preferred nonmedical term for rhinoplasty is "nose reshaping."

Which age groups typically seek rhinoplasty?

Rhinoplasty has been performed on people aged fourteen to seventy who can generally be categorized into three groups.

- Adolescents and young adults, ages fourteen to twenty-two. The impact of cosmetic surgery on this group is explored in Chapter Fifteen.
- People in their midthirties. This group is comprised primarily of working parents who have saved enough money to undergo an operation they have desired most of their lives.
- The over-fifty crowd whose noses have gotten bigger or started to droop with age. They are living proof that nose cartilage continues to grow and change, albeit very slowly, throughout life. Even

people who had an attractive nose through their fourth and fifth decades can develop an unattractive cartilage overgrowth (a bulbous nose) or loose, drooping skin (a hooked nose) as they enter their retirement years. As a result, older patients typically want rhinoplasty just to contour the tip or shorten the nose, comparatively minor procedures. In these cases, rhinoplasty is conceptually similar to facial rejuvenation procedures such as laser peels and eye-lid-lifts.

How popular is rhinoplasty compared with other types of cosmetic surgery?

According to the American Society of Plastic and Re-constructive Surgeons, almost 36,000 rhinoplasties were performed in the United States in 1994, making nose re-shaping one of the top five cosmetic procedures. Next to hair transplants, rhinoplasty is the most common aesthetic surgery among men, and the number-one cosmetic proce-dure among people aged thirty-four and younger.

Why do people seek rhinoplasty?

The simple answer is they are displeased with one or more aspects of their nose. But researchers have found that the psychological profile of rhinoplasty patients is radically different from that of other cosmetic surgery patients. Peo-ple who seek face-lifts, liposuction, or laser peels are ba-sically looking for a younger version of themselves. Rhinoplasty patients, whether they realize it or not, are looking to transform their appearances to a large or small degree. Because that transformation can have an enormous impact on an individual's self-image and self-esteem, rhi-noplasty candidates must be thoroughly screened, both medically and psychologically. The surgeon must be totally convinced before operating that the patient is emotionally stable and has realistic expectations.

Kathy, an actress/model who developed a bump on her

nose after a car accident in 1992, thought nothing of it for three years. Then she saw her profile in a photograph that appeared in a fashion magazine. "I thought to myself, 'Oh my God, my nose looks huge,'" she recalls. "It really bothered me. I became extremely conscious of camera angles."

Kathy was a good candidate for rhinoplasty because she did not expect a new nose to help her get modeling jobs or become a superstar. No one who hired her seemed to care about the bump to begin with. She was simply trying to improve her own comfort level in front of the camera.

During your rhinoplasty consultation, expect the surgeon to ask several questions regarding your motivation, particularly if you are over twenty-five or male. People over twenty-five have lived with their nose for many years and must be mentally healthy enough to cope with such a radical change. Research suggests that male rhinoplasty candidates tend to put too much stake in their operation, and as a result, face an elevated risk for future psychiatric disorders. Men must understand that having their nose reshaped will not save a failing marriage, enhance their sexual performance, help them get dates, make them feel more secure, or change their basic personality. Having rhinoplasty can even backfire. Consider the man who blames his lousy love life on his unattractive nose. If his love life fails to improve after surgery, he no longer has his nose as an excuse. Realizing his life is pretty much the same after rhinoplasty, he may vent feelings of unhappiness, anger or frustration toward his surgeon instead of working to discover the real root of his problem.

The best male rhinoplasty candidate has a stable life and is happily married. He simply has a desire to look better through rhinoplasty without expectations of outward gains.

How has rhinoplasty evolved over the years?

When plastic surgeons began doing a great many rhinoplasties in the 1960s, the trend was the "signature nose."

Surgeons had limited technical options at their disposal, so many patients wound up with similar-looking results.

The 1980s was a decade of reconciliation. Surgeons studied people who had rhinoplasty twenty years prior. These patients' skin had thinned enough over time to reveal the surgical mistakes of the past. There was a consensus among surgeons that a more individualized, scientific approach was needed. New surgical instruments were developed and techniques refined, enabling surgeons to "sculpt" your nose to fit your face instead of giving you someone else's nose. For example, in the 1960s, the most common way to remove a hump from a nose was with a mallet and chisel. Today, a diamond-tipped rasp (file) is used to shave off bone in increments of $1/10$ millimeter.

Paradoxically, the same changes that increased the accuracy and precision of rhinoplasty have also increased the length of operation. The average rhinoplasty lasted an hour or less in the 1960s compared with one-and-a-half to four hours today.

Which types of surgeons perform rhinoplasty?

Plastic surgeons and otolaryngologists (head-and-neck surgeons) do the lion's share of rhinoplasties in this country.

Is there such thing as an "ideal nose?"

The "ideal" nose is different for each individual, although ideal proportions and angles between the nose and the rest of the face are relatively constant. Researchers came up with these constants by measuring many models' faces from every conceivable angle and averaging the measurements. Investigators found, for example, that the angle between the upper lip and the bottom of the nose should be between 90 and 100 degrees on a man. On a woman, that angle should be a bit wider, between 95 and 110 degrees, which means the nose is turned up slightly.

In planning your rhinoplasty, your surgeon examines

dozens of checkpoints to analyze how your nose currently deviates from "ideal." The surgeon considers, among other things, nose length, its projection off your face, its angles, the width of the tip, and nostril size. A patient's height and bone structure also come into play.

This careful analysis translates into dozens of steps in the operation that may or may not be performed. In an effort to create an ideal nose for your face, the surgeon must plan a rhinoplasty much like an architect designs a house to fit on a particular piece of land.

How does a person's height and bone structure help determine a suitable nose shape?

There is no question that a large-boned person should have a larger nose, and vice versa. To give model Cheryl Tiegs's nose to Cher would make the actress/singer look bizarre. A patient's height is important because tall people tend to have "tall" faces that look better with a slightly longer nose.

Do men and women have different preferences as to the shape of their nose?

Society is quite attuned to attractive, petite noses on women, and that is what most women want from surgery. When it comes to men, however, society values a larger, more masculine nose. Big-nosed men who want a much smaller nose should consider actor Tom Cruise. His nose, which is fairly big and has a hump, doesn't seem like the type of nose a man would ask his surgeon to create. But on Tom Cruise, the nose looks great. The same goes for Dustin Hoffman and Al Pacino.

Can rhinoplasty make a small nose bigger?

Prior to the 1980s, almost all rhinoplasties involved nose reduction. Today, with the well-proportioned nose in vogue, surgeons frequently find themselves adding cartilage or bone almost as often as they take it away. In some cases, cartilage removed from one part of the nose can be re-shaped and grafted onto another part of the nose, usually the tip. Graft material also can come from the patient's skull, ear, rib, or nasal septum (the wall that separates the nostrils). The septum is the preferred area for graft material because it is a hidden donor site.

People with a hump in their nose sometimes need a graft to fill in the area where the nose comes off the face between the eyes. Without the graft, the nose begins too low and looks too large. This kind of graft makes the hump look smaller, which means the surgeon won't need to shave off as much to improve proportions.

Are there any medical conditions that would rule me out for surgery?

As with any aesthetic surgical procedure, rhinoplasty should be avoided by anyone with active or severe medical problems, especially bleeding disorders.

Which anesthesia is used?

Rhinoplasty can be performed under local anesthesia with sedation, or under general anesthesia. There is an argument that general anesthesia is actually safer because the airway is protected by a breathing tube. Patients under sedation may have difficulty coughing up blood that can drip down the throat during surgery.

Cocaine is another anesthetic often used during rhino-plasty. Cocaine is both an anesthetic drug and very strong vasoconstrictor. In addition to blocking pain receptors, it shrinks blood vessels and membranes, which minimizes blood loss. Rhinoplasty is one of cocaine's few legal medical uses, although many surgeons have stopped using it because of its high potential for complications, such as irregular heart rhythms.

How is rhinoplasty performed?

There are two surgical methods available to the surgeon: the traditional closed technique, where all the incisions are inside the nostrils; and the newer open technique, where an external incision is made on the "columella" (skin bridge separating the nostrils) and connects to longer internal incisions. The open technique allows the surgeon to lift up the nose skin to get a better view of inner structures. Additional incisions at the bottom of each nostril are made if your nostrils are to be narrowed.

More and more plastic surgeons are turning to the open technique for difficult cases, such as repeat rhinoplasties or correction of twisted or asymmetrical noses. The scar left from the open method is usually extremely difficult to see once it fades.

Through internal or external incisions, the surgeon does any number of procedures such as contouring the tip, shortening the nose, removing a hump, narrowing the nose by making cuts in the bone, and grafting cartilage.

The open technique takes a bit longer but offers a greater degree of accuracy, which increases the chances of a good result, particularly when the surgeon has not done too many rhinoplasties. Which technique a surgeon prefers depends on his or her training and experience.

Should the surgeon also operate on my septum to prevent breathing problems that might arise from rhinoplasty?

Absolutely not. The septum is the nose's most important structural support. It is ridiculous to weaken it for any reason other than to correct a documented breathing obstruction or to harvest cartilage for grafting.

Is rhinoplasty a particularly difficult operation to perform?

Yes. In fact it's considered *the* most difficult procedure in aesthetic plastic surgery. For one thing, nose cartilage is very difficult to work with. To further complicate matters, the surgeon operates upside down and backwards through tiny incisions, usually made inside the nostrils.

The surgeon faces a great number of variables, not the least of which is how a patient will heal. It is impossible to predict how scar tissue and bony callous formation might affect the operation's end result. Precision, therefore, is far more important in rhinoplasty than in, say, liposuction. A tiny difference in circumference from one thigh to the other is not noticeable. However, if the shape, or convexity, of the nose is off by just a half-millimeter, the defect is visible from across a room.

Appreciating the complexity and delicacy of this operation should make you wary of any surgeon who advertises the "fifteen-minute rhinoplasty." It takes fifteen minutes just to draw guidelines on the nose before surgery and another fifteen minutes to drape the patient and for the surgeon to wash his or her hands.

Can rhinoplasty be repeated if necessary?

Yes. Rhinoplasty actually has a high redo rate. Ten to 20 percent of rhinoplasty patients require secondary procedures to compensate for scarring and bone callouses that make their new nose less attractive than it could be. Patients must wait six months to a year for all the swelling to go down before having a second nose-reshaping operation. Otherwise, residual swelling several months after surgery might be mistaken for a permanent hump.

Some plastic surgeons are unwilling to do a repeat rhinoplasty because the level of difficulty triples with these operations. A redo rhinoplasty might be compared to carving a potato encased in cement. These operations are so difficult that there are a few plastic surgeons who actually specialize in redo rhinoplasty.

Fortunately, more than 85 percent of rhinoplasty patients are pleased with their new noses even if they acknowledge that they are not perfect. Of those who have repeat rhinoplasties, some are generally satisfied but want more improvement; others are downright unhappy with their new noses and want them changed again.

Are there any circumstances under which medical insurance would cover my operation?

Unless your nose is broken or was deformed since birth, rhinoplasty is purely cosmetic. Any doctor who attempts to persuade your insurer to reimburse you for this operation is flirting with insurance fraud, a felony.

Medical insurance may cover a related procedure called "septal reconstruction" if a deviated septum is causing a breathing obstruction. A diagnosis of a deviated septum means the wall between your nostrils is slightly off-center. Ninety-five percent of the population has a deviated septum, but only a tiny percentage of deviated septums cause breathing problems. Septal reconstruction can be done in the same operation as rhinoplasty, but it is a different procedure and carries a separate surgeon's fee of $2,000 to $3,000. In many of these cases, an otolaryngologist teams up with a plastic surgeon for the septal reconstruction and rhinoplasty, respectively.

If breathing is impaired, often it is possible to remove part of the "turbinates" in the nose. This bony and soft tissue material often blocks breathing, and its removal is simpler and cheaper than septal surgery.

How much is rhinoplasty?

Surgeons' fees range from about $3,500 to $10,000, depending on the extent of surgery to be done and whether a graft is needed. You will be charged another $1,000 to $2,500 for the operating room and at least $300 an hour for an anesthesiologist.

Will rhinoplasty alter the pitch of my singing or speaking voice?

This is exceedingly unlikely although theoretically possible if bones in the nose wind up blocking a portion of the airway after surgery.

Where is rhinoplasty performed?

Nose reshaping is same-day surgery that can be done in an operating room in the doctor's office, surgicenter, or hospital.

Can rhinoplasty be coupled with other cosmetic procedures?

Yes. It can be performed in conjunction with a face-lift, eyelid-lift, or related facial cosmetic procedure, including a chemical or laser peel.

What will I look like immediately after surgery?

Usually the nose is protected by a splint made of plaster or fiberglass material. Depending on the extent of your surgery, you may or may not have gauze packing in both nostrils to prevent nosebleeds and hold the repositioned internal structures in place.

You will probably have significant swelling and bruises around the central portion of your face. Swelling and bruising may affect your lower and upper eyelids, as well. You will probably be unable to breathe through your nose, and there will be a slight but continuous oozing of blood for about five to fifteen hours after the operation. A drip pad worn under the nose catches the oozing blood.

What will I feel after surgery?

Despite the distortions on their face, most patients experience surprisingly little pain or discomfort.

Will I need an overnight hospital stay or nursing care after surgery?

No. You will need a family member or close friend to help you through the first night, but nursing care is not necessary.

How much down time will I need?

Most patients won't go out in public for almost two weeks after surgery.

What happens during the healing process?

The packing in your nose comes out one to three days after surgery, and the splint and stitches are removed in five to seven days. It takes about three days for the swelling to begin going down. Seventy-five percent of the swelling goes away in two to three weeks, and ninety percent is gone in three months. The remainder of the swelling can take up to a year to completely subside. Try to reserve final judgment on your new nose until after that time.

Is there anything I can do to shorten the healing phase?

Keep fingers and cotton swabs out of your nostrils, and don't blow your nose for a minimum of three weeks after surgery to prevent nosebleeds. Nosebleeds, a major risk factor in the immediate postoperative period, occur in up to 5 percent of rhinoplasty patients.

What other risks and complications are associated with rhinoplasty?

Rhinoplasty patients risk blood clots in the legs or lungs, heart attacks, bad reactions to anesthesia, and death. All these outcomes are extremely rare but possible with any type of major surgery. Rhinoplasty also carries a small risk of postoperative infection and bleeding. About 1 percent of rhinoplasty patients develop breathing problems as a result of surgery.

The risk for aesthetic problems is higher. Ten to 20 percent of patients have various cosmetic deformities, such as a residual hump, bump, asymmetry, collapse of the nose (when the septum has been weakened), arching nostrils, or "parrot beak," also known as "polly beak" (where abnormal fullness forms above the tip).

Does rhinoplasty affect the skin's sensitivity to ultraviolet light?

Yes. Any skin that has been lifted (through a closed or open rhinoplasty) has an increased susceptibility to sun damage and frostbite for the first six months after surgery. To play it safe, wear a sunblock such as zinc oxide on your nose when you go outdoors during the day, and cover your nose with a scarf or neck warmer when skiing and ice-skating for the first year.

How long will the results of my nose reshaping last?

Changes made during rhinoplasty are permanent, but the shape of your nose will continue to evolve. Gradual thinning of the skin and underlying fat eventually will reveal facets of cartilage underneath. Nose cartilage will continue to grow and thicken, and your skin may stretch out and droop as you get older.

Will it be very obvious to other people that I've had a nose job?

That depends on how drastic the changes are. Teenagers tend to want more significant changes, and people can't help but notice (see Chapter Fifteen). Most adult rhinoplasty patients request subtle changes that give their nose a more youthful appearance. Heather said the amount of cartilage removed during her rhinoplasty was so limited that her own parents didn't notice when she visited them less than a week after surgery. ''My eyes were black and blue, so I just covered it with a little makeup,'' she says. Kathy, the actress, said she let her hair grow around the time of her operation, and most friends attributed the change in her appearance to her hairstyle instead of her nose.

It helps to have rhinoplasty at the start of a long vacation. You can detract attention from your anatomical change by altering your hair and makeup.

10

BREASTS BEAUTIFUL, PART ONE

Breast Enlargement Surgery

What motivates women to want bigger breasts?

The vast majority are motivated by the basic desire to look "normal." They want their clothing to fit better, to be able to fill out a shirt or bathing suit appropriately. Patients seeking breast enlargement, or augmentation, typically are flat-chested or small-breasted and wear bras with a B cup or less. Either their breasts never developed to their satisfaction, or their breasts shrunk substantially after they stopped breast-feeding. Self-conscious about their unusually small breasts, most breast-augmentation patients wish to move from an A or AA cup to a B cup, or from a B to a C cup. They want breast implants to attain a more proportional figure and to improve their self-image—not to look like Dolly Parton.

Another group of patients has uneven breasts and wants augmentation to balance them out. In some of these cases, the disparity between breasts is a whole cup size or more. To achieve symmetry, the surgeon can augment one breast and reduce the other, place an implant in just one breast, or use a different-sized implant in each breast. Contrary to the perfectly endowed women pictured in men's magazines, half the female population has asymmetrical breasts. Like women whose breasts are abnormally small, patients unhappy with their asymmetrical breasts seek implant surgery simply to look normal.

Aside from actresses and models, the only other group seeking larger than average breasts are exotic dancers. These women, many of whom already wear a C cup, want to fill a D cup or larger. Their primary motivation is money; dancers with bigger breasts usually get bigger tips.

How popular is breast augmentation compared with other cosmetic procedures?

Since the 1950s, well over two million American women have had their breasts enlarged. Each year in the United States, another 40,000 or so breast-implant operations are performed, making breast augmentation the third most popular form of cosmetic surgery on women, after liposuction and eyelid-lifts.

What is the history of breast implants?

Breast-augmentation surgery began in the 1950s, when various types of rubber and plastic implants were used. These early implants all resulted in hard breasts and other problems. More disastrous results occurred in the early 1960s, when doctors attempted to enlarge breasts with injections of liquid silicone. Injected silicone would travel throughout the chest wall, trigger infection, and, in many cases, lead to mastectomies.

Also during the 1960s, an implant made of silicone gel encased in a flexible, silicone-rubber bag was introduced. The silicone-gel implant represented a major advance over previous implants because it resulted in softer, more natural-feeling breasts. Another type of implant, the same silicone-rubber bag filled with saline (saltwater) was available but hardly ever used because saline was heavier and felt less natural than silicone gel.

In the 1970s, implant manufacturers made a thinner silicone rubber bag so the gel implants would feel even more like normal breast tissue. Later, a bag made of polyurethane-coated silicone was tried. Breasts augmented with these implants felt softer still. But, by the 1980s, plastic surgeons realized that silicone gel could diffuse through the thinner bags, and they feared the same might happen with the polyurethane bag. To prevent these so-called "gel bleeds," the implant bag was made more durable around 1985. Two years later, silicone-gel encased in a textured, as opposed to smooth-walled, bag was introduced. This new, rough bag resulted in less scar tissue forming around the implant.

The silicone-gel implant was plunged into controversy in the late 1980s when thousands of women began alleging that their implants were making them sick. These women— most of whom had breast-augmentation surgery prior to 1985—blamed their gel bleeds for an array of symptoms and diseases, including rheumatoid arthritis, scleroderma, fatigue, dry mouth, bladder problems, memory loss, joint pain, and cancer. In 1991, a California woman received $7.3 million in a lawsuit against one implant manufacturer, Dow Corning Corporation. The following year, the U.S. Food and Drug Administration (FDA), which regulates all medical devices, placed a moratorium on silicone-gel implants. A torrent of lawsuits against implant makers followed.

Despite the FDA's action and patients' claims of injury, scientists have been unable to link silicone gel implants with any unusual symptoms or illnesses. Several reports published in the *New England Journal of Medicine* in 1995 and 1996 looked at thousands of women with silicone implants—some intact, some ruptured—and found no increase in the incidence of headaches, hair loss, arthritis-type diseases, leukemia, or any other medical disorder. Deeming the implants exonerated, European nations and most other countries have since lifted their bans. In the United States, silicone-gel implants continue to be outlawed. The only women who may legally receive silicone-gel implants are those participating in clinical studies that continue to evaluate implant safety.

After a temporary falloff in the number of women undergoing breast augmentation, the operation's popularity is now close to where it was before the silicone gel controversy began. Saline-filled implants are the only type of breast implant widely available in this country today. They come in smooth and textured bags—all made of rubberized silicone.

Are saline-filled implants safe?

While all forms of implant surgery carry inherent risks, there are no known illnesses associated with saline-filled implants, in particular. If the bag leaks, your body merely gets a "drink" of saltwater.

Moreover, the silicone in the rubber bag cannot migrate around the chest wall the way liquid silicone did. There can be microscopic migration of silicone molecules from the bag to surrounding tissues, including lymph nodes, but this has never been shown to be harmful. Indeed, silicone is ubiquitous in nature and manmade devices, such as nipples on baby bottles, coatings on hypodermic needles, pacemakers, artificial hips, artificial finger joints, and various other implants. Because hypodermic needles are lubricated with silicone, insulin-dependent diabetics have extremely high levels of silicone in their bodies. If silicone were truly poisonous to humans, there would be epidemics of silicone-related diseases around the world. In addition, silicone is a legal food additive and is a component of many drugs, including antacids.

What are the surgical risks of breast augmentation?

Like other types of surgery, breast augmentation carries a small risk of bleeding and infection. If breast tissue around the implants becomes infected, the devices must be removed and cannot be replaced for at least six months after the infection clears up. There is a chance of visible scars forming with breast augmentation, as with any surgery.

What are the possible long-term complications of breast augmentation?

All breast implants trigger scar formation, which walls off the implant from surrounding tissue. Making scar tissue is the human body's way of protecting itself against foreign objects, be it a breast implant, shard of glass, or splinter of wood. Historically, up to 40 percent of patients made so much scar tissue around their implants that it led to firmer than desirable breasts. However, with the new textured implant bags, only about 10 percent of patients are expected to develop firm breasts. This phenomenon, known as "capsular contracture," bothers some women more than others. In about 5 percent of patients, the scar tissue squeezes the implant enough to distort the appearance of the breasts. In 3 percent of patients, the scar tissue presses the implant against the ribs and nerves, causing pain. The only remedy in these cases is to remove or replace the implants and break up the scar tissue.

Asymmetrical breasts is another possible complication. One breast might end up slightly higher or lower than the other, or off to the side. Patients can experience a decrease or increase in sensation of the nipple, breast skin, or both. In some cases, you can feel the implant by touching your breast. A ridge, also known as "rippling," may be visible. So-called "sloshing" of a saline implant is a well-known yet extremely rare complication. It results only when the surgeon mistakenly leaves air in the saline-filled implant, which is filled with fluid after it is placed in the breast.

The position of your nipple should not change following breast augmentation.

Can breast implants obscure mammography images?

Unequivocally, the answer is yes. The exact percentage of breast tissue obscured by implants is debatable and differs according to breast x-ray equipment and technique. But there is no dispute that implants obscure at least a small percentage of tissue and perhaps up to 40 percent or more. One in eight American women develops breast cancer. Mammography can detect these cancers when they are highly curable—up to two years before a tumor is large enough to be felt. If you are unlucky enough to have a malignancy in a region hidden by your breast implant, the ultimate consequence of having larger breasts could be your death. Many women decide against having breast implants because of the mammography issue. Women with implants should tell their radiologists before having a mammogram. The technician may be able to manipulate the breast during the scan to achieve the best possible image.

Aside from avoiding breast implants altogether, there are two, but radical, ways around the mammography limitation. One is to have your implants removed at age forty, when a baseline mammography is recommended for most women. The other is to have an MRI (magnetic resonance imaging) scan instead of the traditional low-dose breast x-ray. MRI is far more sensitive than x-ray mammography and can "see" around the implant, but it costs ten times as much. While MRI may someday become the standard for mammography, it is unlikely that insurance will pay for MRI unless its price comes down substantially.

Women with a strong family history of breast cancer should be discouraged from having their breasts enlarged. Be concerned about the physician who is willing to do the surgery on you if breast cancer has stricken two or more immediate blood relatives, such as a mother and sister.

Will having breast implants impede my ability to do a proper breast self-exam?

Since the implant is placed under the breast tissue, it should not make a difference unless you are one of the women who develops an extreme amount of scarring around the implant.

Aside from a family history of breast cancer, what other situations would make me unsuitable for breast implants?

Diabetics and women with other general health problems should avoid breast augmentation, as should anyone taking steroids to treat various medical disorders.

Women with significant drooping of the breasts are often better served by the breast-lift operation (see Chapter Eleven). Breast implants in these individuals might accentuate the droopiness.

You should also consider psychological and emotional factors when deciding whether to augment your breasts. If you want larger breasts solely to please your husband or boyfriend, take pause. Bigger breasts will not make you a better lover or change the nature of your relationship. If you have deep-seated marital problems, more cleavage won't solve them.

What is the age range of women receiving breast implants?

Breast augmentation can be performed on girls as young as seventeen, as long as the surgeon is sure that all growth and natural breast development are completed. The teen must be several years beyond puberty and as tall or taller than her parents.

The oldest women receiving implants are generally in their forties, usually because they lost breast volume after having children. This loss in volume stems from pressure that expanding milk-producing tissue placed on fatty tissue during pregnancy and breast-feeding. It is well established that fat cells are destroyed under pressure. The result is small, drooping breasts that can be improved substantially through breast augmentation, a breast-lift (see Chapter Eleven), or both.

How is implant size determined prior to surgery?

Ultimately, the decision is up to you—with strong counseling from your plastic surgeon. Most women want to get to an average size, a large B cup or small C cup. Most plastic surgeons try to dissuade women from becoming too large. Large breasts can lead to back and neck pain, rashes under the breasts, and bra straps digging into the shoulders (''notching''). These discomforts are the reasons large-breasted women seek reduction surgery (see Chapter Twelve). It is also important to realize that only your cup size will change. If you currently wear a 34A bra, you will wear a 34B after surgery, not a 36B.

Is it possible to know how my breasts will look after surgery?

A completely accurate prediction is impossible, but you can get an approximate estimation of what your breast size will be. One popular way is to bring to your consultation a bra you think you want to fit into. Don't bring in a push-up bra or a barely there lacy number you bought at Victoria's Secret. Bring in a full-cup bra your immigrant grandmother would be proud of. Put on the bra and stand in front of a mirror. Have your surgeon put progressively larger implants in the cups, beginning with implants that are too small and ending up with ones that are too big for your body structure. It will become apparent which size is appropriate for you. Chances are you will be happiest with a midsize implant.

Will my breasts feel heavier after surgery?

There is no question that your breasts will feel heavier, especially with saline-filled implants, which are basically water balloons. (On a volume basis, silicone gel is lighter.) For example, an average saline-filled implant big enough to boost you from an A to a small C cup weighs slightly more than half a pound—a total of 1.1 pounds for two implants. Although your breasts will never feel completely natural, the added weight will be less noticeable over time.

What is the cost of breast-augmentation surgery?

Surgeons' fees range from $3,000 to $5,000. You will be charged an additional $1,000 or so for a pair of implants. Anesthesia fees run from about $800 to $1,200, and the operating room will cost you another $1,000 to $2,000, depending on whether you use a hospital or office-based facility. The procedure is normally done on an outpatient basis.

How long does the operation take?

Breast augmentation with saline-filled implants takes about two-and-a-half hours, slightly longer than augmentation with silicone-gel implants requires. The reason is that the saline implants must first be filled and tested for leaks, deflated, positioned in the breasts, and finally refilled with saline through its valve before the incision is closed.

What kind of anesthesia is used?

Breast augmentation is usually performed under general anesthesia, although it can be done under local anesthesia with sedation. Nausea and other risks are associated with general anesthesia, but there have been rare cases of punctured lungs when local anesthesia was injected into the breast area.

How long will the incision be?

Because the saline implant is deflated during insertion, a relatively small incision—just over an inch long—is usually all that is needed. Incision size is a significant advantage over the silicone-gel implant, which required a two-inch-long incision.

Where is the incision made?

There are four possible sites. The most common is in the skin crease under the breast. The scar resulting from this incision is not visible unless you are lying down naked.

The second is the lower edge of areola, the pigmented region around the nipple. Like the under-the-breast incision, the areola entry point affords the surgeon great accuracy in placing the implant. However, the scar can be seen when you are standing, sitting, or lying down naked.

The last two, and least common, incisions are used with the aid of an endoscope (see Chapter One). An armpit incision is possible but leaves a fairly long scar that can be seen whenever you lift your arms while wearing a bathing suit or sleeveless shirt. Endoscopic implant placement through the armpit incision also carries a higher risk of asymmetry and injury to nerves and blood vessels. Recently, the implants have been placed through the belly-button incision, which leaves a hidden scar, but this is seldom used because of the great distance the implant must travel to reach its destination. Implant manufacturers may not warranty any implant placed through the belly button because its chance of being damaged is greater than with other techniques.

Endoscopic breast augmentation does have its advantages. It keeps incisions off the breasts, and it allows surgeons to create a pocket for the implant more efficiently and control bleeding much more effectively. Endoscopy is not offered for breast augmentation by every plastic surgeon, but there are some who are highly skilled in this technique.

Your surgeon may let you choose from two or more incision sites. It behooves you to ask your surgeon which he or she is most comfortable with.

What happens after the incision is made?

The surgeon carefully creates a pocket in the breast large enough to accommodate the inflated implant. The pocket can be made either above or below the pectoralis muscle, the muscle in the chest responsible for drawing the arm forward and inward. The implant, with its attached filling tube, is carefully placed in the pocket. A predetermined amount of saline (typically 250 cc) is injected into the implant through the filling tube, displacing any air remaining in the implant. The tube is removed, automatically sealing the valve on the implant bag. The incision is closed with sutures and dressed.

Is it better to place the implant under or over the pectoralis muscle?

Each has its advantages, but there are different considerations for different women. Women under age thirty generally prefer to have their breast implants above the muscle. This is especially important for active, athletic women who want to wear skintight leotards or bathing suits. If the implant is under the muscle, the breast will visibly flatten each time she flexes her pectoralis.

Older women, particularly those with droopy breasts, tend to prefer the under-the-muscle placement. This technique is more conducive to breast-lift surgery, should it be needed. More importantly, under-the-muscle placement allows slightly more breast tissue to be seen on a mammogram.

How long is the recovery period after breast augmentation?

If your implants are over the muscle, you can probably go back to work in about five days, unless your job involves physical labor. You will need two weeks before returning to work if your implants are under the muscle.

How much pain should I expect during the healing process?

There will be surprisingly little pain if your implant is over the muscle. However, you should anticipate a fair amount of discomfort if your implants are under muscle. When muscle tissue is cut, it hurts. Your doctor can prescribe medication to help minimize any pain.

How much swelling will I experience?

Quite a bit. After surgery, your breasts will be about 25 percent larger than they will be ultimately. It will take about three weeks for the swelling to subside enough so you can shop for your new bra wardrobe. It takes about three months until the swelling is completely gone.

Can I go braless after surgery?

Wearing a bra is required as a surgical support for the first month or so after your operation. Afterward, wearing a bra is strongly recommended to decrease the rate of drooping.

Can the surgery be redone if the implants are placed too high, asymmetrically, or seem too large or too small?

There are techniques that can be used to reposition the implants through the use of pressure garments. If the asymmetry persists beyond several months, however, your surgeon may need to reopen the incisions in one or both breasts to fix the problem.

Are most women satisfied with their new breasts?

Breast augmentation has a very high satisfaction rate, in the neighborhood of 98 or 99 percent. Most women who wind up with firm breasts are willing to accept it as a consequence of surgery.

How soon after surgery can I exercise?

Avoid exercise for the first three weeks after surgery. Over the next three weeks, you may gradually get back to your normal exercise routine. Be sure to wear a supportive sports bra while exercising.

Should I massage my breasts after surgery?

If your implants have a textured bag, massage is not recommended or necessary to keep the breasts soft. If you have smooth-shelled implants (which cost about $200 less than textured ones), massaging your breasts for several minutes each day will help keep the implant pocket as large as possible, which reduces the risk of firmness and distortion later on.

How long will my implants last?

Saline-filled implants are not considered lifetime devices. They maintain breast enlargement until they deflate. When that happens is anyone's guess. Statistically, 1 percent of all saline implants put in this year will deflate over the ensuing twelve months. After ten years, 10 percent of this year's implants will have deflated. You will know your implant has probably deflated if the size or shape of your breast changes or if you experience breast pain.

Should my saline implants be removed if they deflate?

Breast distortion and pain are indications for implant removal. Unfortunately, the statistics are grim when it comes to replacing the deflated implants with new ones: About 50 percent of women who had trouble with their first implants will experience similar problems with subsequent implants. Some people simply cannot tolerate breast implants. Most sensible plastic surgeons will give the patient one or two tries after the original placement. If problems continue, the implants should be permanently removed. There is no way to predict which patients will have problems; there is no correlation between how scar tissue behaves on the skin and how internal scar tissue behaves.

What will my breasts look like if my implants are removed?

Chances are your breasts will look smaller and droopier than they did before surgery. Your surgeon may be able to return a semblance of attractiveness by performing a breast-lift operation.

Will I be able to breast-feed after receiving implants?

You should still be able to breast-feed with no harm to you or your baby. Studies have found no increase in breast-milk silicone levels among women with implants compared to women with no implants. As alluded to earlier, silicone is the most abundant chemical on Earth. Everyone has some level of silicone in their bodies, with no adverse impact on health.

Will my significant other notice the difference?

If a person never saw or felt your bare breasts before surgery, he may not notice you have implants unless he is familiar with the feeling. If you keep the lights low, he may not even notice the scar.

Are there new types of implants on the horizon?

Yes. A variety of researchers are attempting to develop implants that feel natural like silicone gel but won't obscure mammograms. Among the implant fillers being examined are peanut oil and other fatty substances, which would be digested by the body if the bag ruptures. Studies of new implants are probably two or three years away from completion, but the FDA is unlikely to be quick on the trigger when it comes to approving them for widespread use.

At least one new implant, called the Trilucent implant, is already in use in the United Kingdom, according to the implant's manufacturer, the Collagen Corporation. According to the company, the Trilucent implant is "designed to be less of a barrier to successful mammography" than either saline-filled or silicone-gel implants.

11

BREASTS BEAUTIFUL, PART TWO

Breast-Lift Surgery

Why do my breasts droop?

Like every other part of your body, breast tissue changes as you age. It looses some elasticity and fat, and droops or sags under the force of gravity. The nipples, which normally point out and slightly up, gradually descend and begin to point downward. (If you notice a significant change or asymmetry in your nipples, it could be a sign of breast disease. See your gynecologist or internist immediately.)

Aside from natural aging, there are other forces that make the breasts droop. Many mothers find that their breasts shrink as their children grow. Because their breasts were once larger, particularly during pregnancy and breast-feeding, these women may develop significant drooping in their late thirties and forties. Women who gain and lose a large amount of weight also tend to have drooping breasts because their breast skin has been stretched.

The severity of breast droop depends on several factors, including your genetic profile, the weight of your breasts and overall body weight, how many pounds you gained during pregnancy, and how much time you spend out of a bra. People who like to go braless tend to have droopier breasts; that includes women who sleep without a bra. Unless your breasts are supported when you are lying down, they hang over your body, stretching out the breast skin.

How can I tell whether I need a breast-lift or breast implants?

Ask yourself this fundamental question: "Is my problem volume or shape?" If you are happy with your appearance in a bra, you probably have an adequate amount of breast tissue and may benefit from a breast-lift, or mastopexy. If you do not like the way your breasts look in or out of a bra, you may be a candidate for breast augmentation, possibly combined with a breast-lift. Your plastic surgeon can help you decide which procedure is most appropriate.

What is a breast-lift?

A breast-lift is a surgical procedure designed to restore a more youthful appearance to sagging, droopy breasts. To accomplish this goal, the plastic surgeon removes excess skin, repositions the nipple, and redrapes and tightens the remaining skin to support the breast.

Must the nipple be completely removed before it is repositioned?

To preserve nipple sensation and function, most plastic surgeons no longer completely detach the nipple. The nipple (including the areola) is completely freed up from surrounding skin but is left attached to underlying tissue, including milk ducts, blood supply, and nerve endings. The nipple is sewn into a more appropriate position on the lifted breast, generally higher than it was previously.

Is it possible to predict how I will look after a mastopexy?

It is impossible to know precisely how you will look, but you can get a general idea by looking in the mirror while wearing a push-up bra. Your cup size won't change, but your nipples will be lifted to the level of the crease underneath your breasts.

What does mastopexy cost?

The plastic surgeon's fee ranges from about $3,000 to $6,000, depending on the surgical approach. Anesthesiology and operating room fees also vary according to the length of surgery, which can run anywhere from one-and-a-half to four hours.

Where is mastopexy performed?

Mastopexy can be performed in a hospital, office-based, or free-standing operating room. It is usually done as an outpatient, although an overnight stay may be necessary when several breast incisions are made.

What kind of anesthesia is used?

This procedure is usually done under general anesthesia.

Where are the incisions made?

There are three main mastopexy techniques, each requiring a different set of incisions. The first technique, designed for women whose nipples have not descended significantly, requires one continuous incision around the areola. The second technique features a "lollipop" incision: The same cut is made around the areola, but it connects to a vertical incision down the lower half of the breast to the chest wall. The third and most effective technique utilizes the lollipop incision plus a one- to five-inch-long incision made horizontally underneath the breast. This technique leaves the most scarring but achieves the best results.

All the techniques involve cutting away excess skin and tightening the remaining skin to lift up the breasts. The extent to which the nipple is repositioned varies from patient to patient.

How much pain will I experience?

Mastopexy is not a particularly painful operation since no muscle is cut. Any discomfort you experience can usually be controlled with acetaminophen with codeine for a day or two following surgery.

When do the stitches come out?

Skin stitches usually come out by the seventh day after surgery. You will also have a second layer of stitches underneath the skin, but those will dissolve over time.

How much down time will I need?

Most mastopexy patients need to take off at least a week or two before returning to work or their normal routine.

Is there anything I can do to promote healing after surgery?

Maintain a good, balanced diet, and don't sleep facedown for at least a month after surgery. If you sleep on your stomach, the weight of your body could split open the incisions.

What risks are associated with mastopexy?

There is a small chance of infection or bleeding. The nipple is a little numb in 1 to 4 percent of mastopexy patients. Nipple numbness can be temporary or permanent. There also may be some numbness of the breast skin, but this is usually temporary.

Ninety-five percent of patients eventually heal with thin, flat, light-colored scars. Some patients develop wider scars, and about 5 percent wind up with permanent red, raised scars.

If you exercise or sleep facedown too soon after surgery, you run the risk of opening your incisions. Diabetics are also at a higher than average risk for this complication.

If you smoke, the results of mastopexy can be disastrous. Lifting and placing the skin under tension reduces its blood supply. Despite that punishment, the skin usually does just fine—except in smokers, who have diminished blood flow to begin with. Parts of their breast skin and nipples may not survive the surgery. When tissue dies, it is replaced by scars, which can result in disfigurement severe enough to require reconstructive surgery later on. For this reason, many plastic surgeons simply refuse to perform breast-lifts, or any type of lifting procedure, on smokers.

Do the scars that result from this procedure dissuade many women from having mastopexy?

Yes. Like candidates for tummy tucks and face-lifts, women exploring breast-lift surgery should see pictures of former patients' scars before making a final decision. Mastopexy is a purely aesthetic operation with no therapeutic benefit. Many women concerned enough with the appearance of their bare breasts are unwilling to tolerate that much scarring. Fortunately, the scars cannot be seen under sleeveless blouses and bathing-suit tops, unless the bathing suit reveals the bottom portion of the breasts.

What kind of bra should I wear after surgery?

A very supportive bra, preferably one without underwires, should be worn for at least a month after surgery and, ideally, forever. If you have gone through the trouble and expense of lifting your breasts, you'll probably want to do everything possible to prevent future drooping. Wearing a good bra, even when you sleep, is a major step in that direction. The bra should open in the front so that arm motion and contortion are minimized when dressing and undressing.

How long will it be before I can exercise comfortably?

Generally you should do no exercise for three weeks after surgery. Over the next three weeks, you can gradually build up to your previous level of physical activity.

Will my breasts look bigger after surgery?

Breasts do look to be larger and have more cleavage after mastopexy, especially when you are wearing a low-cut shirt or dress. But that is an illusion. There will be more volume in the upper portion of your breasts, but your bra size will stay the same. The effect of the surgery is almost like wearing a permanent, invisible pushup bra.

Will my breasts be symmetrical after surgery?

No two breasts going into surgery are perfectly symmetrical, and having exact symmetry after surgery is unlikely. Fortunately, slight discrepancies in breast appearance are not noticeable or bothersome to the vast majority of patients. There are, of course, exceptions. One mastopexy patient took a ruler to her breasts and was distressed to discover that one nipple was 1 millimeter higher than the other. If your expectations of perfection are that extreme, you are unlikely to be fully satisfied after a breast-lift or any cosmetic surgical procedure.

What is the life span of this operation?

Your breast-lift should last five to ten years, maybe longer. Like any cosmetic procedure that lifts stretched-out tissue, mastopexy cannot stop the aging process. Aging resumes the day after surgery. How long your breast-lift lasts depends on how much weight you gain and lose, how often you wear a bra, how supportive that bra is, and whether you become pregnant. Most women hold off having a mastopexy until after giving birth to their last child.

If I should become pregnant after a mastopexy, will I be able to breast-feed my baby?

You should be able to breast-feed since the milk ducts are never detached from the nipple during surgery. If a postoperative infection sets in, however, it can destroy your ability to breast-feed. Remember that pregnancy and breast-feeding could lead to droopy breasts once again.

Does mastopexy hamper mammography or breast self-exams?

It should not. There will be swelling for three to six months after the operation, making it uncomfortable or painful to examine your breasts manually or undergo mammography. If you are at the age when mammography is important, the scan should be done prior to your breast-lift operation and repeated after surgery to document surgery-caused changes.

What percentage of mastopexy patients are pleased with the outcome of their surgery?

Most women who knew beforehand what their scars would look like are pleased with their breast-lifts. As with other cosmetic procedures, the happiest mastopexy patients are the ones who are prepared, not surprised.

❖ 12 ❖

BREASTS BEAUTIFUL, PART THREE

Breast-Reduction Surgery

What usually motivates women to have breast-reduction surgery?

There are both cosmetic and physical reasons for having your breast size reduced. The most common cosmetic complaint by women wanting "reduction mammoplasty" is that their clothes don't fit properly over their excessively large breasts. This problem may or may not be accompanied by such physical symptoms as upper and lower back pain, neck pain, poor posture, notches in the shoulders caused by bra straps digging into the skin, rashes underneath the breasts from chafing, and recurrent yeast infections under the breasts.

How old is the typical breast-reduction patient?

Breast-reduction surgery has been performed on women in their late teens to middle age, but the vast majority are either college-aged or in their late thirties to early forties.

Leslie, a clinical social worker, had her breasts reduced at age thirty-one, a year after the birth of her second child. "I was uncomfortable with my breasts ever since they popped out in eighth grade," Leslie explains. "But I didn't learn about the operation until someone had it when I was a junior in college. Ever since then, that was my goal."

Is it possible to predict how I'll look after surgery?

Your surgeon aims to create a breast size you will be happy with, but reduction mammoplasty is not a precise enough operation to guarantee an exact size. Candidates for breast reduction typically wear a D cup or larger, and in most cases, their nipples have migrated downward under the force of gravity. After reduction surgery, your breast size will be small, average or large, depending on what you expressed to your surgeon prior to the operation, and your nipples will be about level with the crease under your breasts. "Small" means anywhere from a large A cup to a small B cup. "Average" ranges from a large B to a small C cup. And "large" is classified as a large C to a small D cup.

Leslie's breast size fluctuated but was always excessive. "At my lowest weight, 106 pounds, I was still a 34DD," she says. When she was nursing her babies, her breast size ballooned to an "H cup." The day she walked into the operating room, Leslie was "busting out of a 38DDD."

Four months after surgery, Leslie was down to a 36C—a difference she calls "astounding."

"It was really unimaginable a few months ago that I could look like this," says Leslie. "I used to have to lift my breasts up to wash, now I go to do it, and there's practically nothing there. This is the best thing I ever did for myself."

What happens during the operation?

The surgeon makes the same three incisions used in the third breast-lifting technique described in the previous chapter: around the areola, vertically from the bottom center of the areola to the crease under the breast, and horizontally curved along the breast crease. This last incision spans almost the entire width of the breast, ending about a half-inch from the midline.

Working through the incisions, the surgeon cuts away excess breast tissue, fat, and skin above and on either side of the nipple. The nipple is raised to a higher position on the breast and sewn into place. The skin is lifted and re-contoured around the remaining breast tissue and sutured into its new position. This phase of the operation is similar to breast-lift surgery (see Chapter Eleven).

Breast tissue that was removed is examined by a pathologist for signs of disease. This precautionary measure is required by law in most states because of the propensity for breast tissue to become cancerous.

Must the nipple be completely detached before it is repositioned?

No. Since the 1970s, most surgeons have performed the procedure with a technique that leaves the nipple attached to underlying breast tissue, including milk ducts, nerve endings, and blood vessels. However, some plastic surgeons still perform a procedure that removes the nipple and re-places it later in the operation as a graft. The reasoning for this is that there is less risk of destruction of the nipple with this technique. Most doctors disagree with that point of view.

The goals of keeping the nipple attached to underlying tissue are to maintain sensation, to enable breast-feeding, and to give the nipple as normal an appearance as possible. These goals are not always met, however. One in three breast-reduction patients ends up with permanent numbness in one or both nipples. Also, there is a small but present danger that the blood supply will be inadequate to keep the nipple alive. If the nipple does not survive, it is replaced by scar tissue, necessitating nipple-reconstruction surgery later on. This happens in 1 to 2 percent of cases.

When grafted, the nipple survives in about 98 percent of cases. However, grafted nipples often scar, become lighter in color, and no longer look natural. There is no sensation in a grafted nipple, and breast-feeding is out of the question.

Is it possible to perform a mammoplasty without repositioning the nipple?

Yes, but circumstances warranting this approach are rare. In almost all instances, excessively large breasts sag so much that the skin stretches and the nipples descend. If the nipples are not repositioned during surgery, they will be too low on the breast.

How does the surgeon know how much breast tissue to remove?

How much skin and tissue to remove is a judgment call by the physician. The more training and experience the surgeon has, the more likely he or she will be to remove the appropriate amount to achieve the breast volume you desire.

Which anesthesia is used?

Breast reductions are almost always performed while the patient is under general anesthesia.

How long does the operation take?

Reduction mammoplasty takes anywhere from three to five hours, depending on the extent of the reduction.

How long is the recovery period?

Most patients experience some pain and discomfort immediately after surgery and require narcotic painkillers for one to two days. Your stitches will be taken out in one to two weeks. You should not lie facedown for at least three weeks. Most patients need one to two weeks off work after reduction mammoplasty. If your job requires physical activity, you should stay home an additional week.

Most of the swelling should go down within a month after surgery, and the rest of the swelling normally disappears in about three months.

Will the scars be visible?

Unfortunately, the scars left by this operation will be obvious when you are disrobed. They are easily hidden by a bra or bathing suit that is not too revealing.

Should I have a mammogram before surgery?

Most plastic surgeons require a mammogram just before and three months after your operation. By comparing the two scans, the doctor can see what changes have occurred as a result of the surgery and where scar tissue has formed. The postoperative breast x-ray becomes your new baseline mammogram to be compared with regularly scheduled future mammograms.

Can mammoplasty improve the accuracy of mammography scans?

In some ways, reading mammograms after breast reductions is easier, and in other ways more difficult. It is easier because there is less breast tissue to examine. It is more difficult because scar tissue stemming from the operation could imitate cancer or obscure a malignant growth. This is why it is vitally important to have a postoperative baseline mammography. Rest assured, this operation in no way causes cancer or makes it more likely.

What does breast-reduction surgery cost?

Surgeons' fees range from about $4,500 to $8,500. The anesthesiologist will charge a minimum of $1,500. A hospital operating room and overnight stay can cost upwards of $5,000. If you have the operation as an outpatient, the operating room fee is $1,600 to $2,000. Patients are charged several hundred dollars more for pathology, mammography, and if necessary, examinations by an orthopedist or other specialist.

Does health insurance cover reduction mammoplasty?

Not as often as in the past. Until the early 1990s, 98 percent of insurers paid for reduction mammoplasty with very few questions asked. All the surgeon needed to do was diagnose a bona fide symptom, such as back pain or rashes under the breasts, or simply state that the breasts are very large and uncomfortable and will lead to physical problems down the line.

Today, only about half of insurance plans cover reduction mammoplasty. Plastic surgeons are being asked to thoroughly document which functional problem or problems the operation will solve. The patient must undergo a thorough evaluation, sometimes by more than one specialist. For example, some insurers require photographs of the patient's bare breasts and a detailed exam by an orthopedic surgeon or neurologist to document that the patient's back pain indeed stems from her oversized breasts and cannot be alleviated in any other way. Some patients are so daunted by these new requirements that they keep postponing the operation or opt out of it. It sometimes seems that the goal of insurance companies is to put up so many "hoops" to jump through that the patient gives up.

Leslie considers herself lucky that her insurer picked up the tab for her operation and overnight hospital stay. "Even if it didn't," she says, "I would have paid for it myself and never had a regret."

Can reduction mammoplasty be performed in an outpatient setting?

To keep the procedure affordable for women who cannot obtain insurance reimbursement, more and more plastic surgeons are doing reduction mammoplasty in outpatient settings—namely office-based operating rooms and free-standing surgicenters. However, many women who have breast reduction require an overnight stay in the hospital, and some need a two-night stay. The most common reason to stay overnight in the hospital is nausea resulting from the long period of time under general anesthesia. A less costly alternative to hospitalization is hiring a visiting nurse to help you through the first twenty-four to forty-eight hours after surgery.

Are there any medical conditions that would rule me out as a candidate for breast reduction?

Cosmetic surgeons prefer patients whose overall health status is good. Most would be extremely reluctant to do reduction mammoplasty on someone with diabetes or high blood pressure.

What risks and complications are associated with breast-reduction surgery?

As with any major surgery, there is a small risk of post-operative infection, bleeding, blood clots in the legs or lungs, or even death. Nausea and vomiting are common occurrences after general anesthesia.

Aside from potential nipple problems discussed earlier, there is a small risk that you will heal with red, thick scars instead of flat, flesh-toned scars. Dark-skinned women tend to heal with scars that are darker than surrounding skin. Diabetics are at a particularly high risk of healing irregularities, and people with uncontrolled or poorly controlled high blood pressure are more likely to have a bleeding problem soon after surgery. All breast-reduction patients risk losing some sensation in the breast skin, which can be temporary or permanent. Skin loss due to inadequate blood flow is another possibility, but this complication is more likely to occur in smokers than nonsmokers.

Impaired breast-feeding is another potential complication. Depending on how much breast tissue was removed, you may be unable to produce enough milk to sustain your baby. If you develop an infection after surgery, or if you have a problem with the blood supply to the nipple, you may be unable to produce milk. More importantly, pregnancy causes the breasts to grow, stretch, and droop again. If you are planning a pregnancy, you may wish to postpone reduction mammoplasty until after you've had all the children you want.

Can I have liposuction to reduce my breast size?

In general, liposuction (see Chapter Thirteen) does not work for breast reduction because the consistency of breast tissue is extremely variable and therefore difficult to remove by fat vacuuming. Some plastic surgeons use liposuction in conjunction with conventional reduction techniques, particularly to remove fatty breast tissue under the arms.

If I am overweight, will the surgeon insist that I lose weight before performing surgery?

If you had smaller breasts before your weight gain, you may be able to shrink your breast size through diet and exercise and save yourself the expense and inconvenience of surgery. However, being overweight does not exclude a woman from having reduction mammoplasty, as long as she isn't morbidly obese. In fact, having breast-reduction surgery may serve as an impetus to losing weight. Leslie was inspired to drop fourteen pounds in the first four months after her operation.

The surgery itself will leave you a pound or two lighter. And you will soon discover how much easier it is to exercise when you have smaller breasts.

Can I go braless after breast-reduction surgery?

Once healing is complete—several months after surgery—you can go braless. However, reduced breasts are still prone to drooping if they are not supported by a bra most of the time. The majority of women who have reduction mammoplasty wear a supportive bra because they want to preserve their new breast shape as long as possible. Some go so far as to wear a bra to sleep.

How long can the results of this operation be expected to last?

Unless you become pregnant, you will have smaller breasts for the rest of your life.

What percentage of women who have breast reduction is satisfied with the results?

This operation enjoys an extremely high satisfaction rate—almost 100 percent—despite the scarring. One gynecologist, Dr. Vrunda Patel of Princeton, New Jersey, remarks that her happiest patients are those who have had breast-reduction surgery. "Their only regret is not having it done sooner," Dr. Patel observes.

Will shrinking my breast size lower my breast-cancer risk?

No. There is absolutely no difference in breast cancer rates among women who have had breast reduction and those who have not. Every cell in the breast has a potential to become malignant. The only way to decrease your breast-cancer risk is to have a double mastectomy, which includes the removal of the nipples and every trace of breast tissue.

Can breast-reduction surgery be redone if I want to go smaller or my breasts or nipples are asymmetrical after surgery?

Touchups after reduction mammoplasty are not particularly common. But if your breasts end up uneven or are still too large, you can safely have followup surgery.

✤ 13 ✤

EASIER THAN DIETING?

Fat Reduction Through Liposuction

What is liposuction?

Liposuction is a surgical procedure by which excess fat is manually broken up and then vacuumed out of the body through a rigid, hollow, blunt-ended tube called a cannula. Cannulas have holes near the ends through which the fat is suctioned. Liposuction is also known as "suction-assisted lipectomy," "liposculpture," and "lipoplasty."

How did liposuction get started?

Liposuction was first described in France in the early 1980s. It was a response to the desire of many people to have excess body fat removed without the enormous scars left by the other body-contouring techniques available at that time.

In the early years of the procedure, many problems were experienced, giving the operation a bad reputation. Liposuction was attempted through as few incisions as possible, giving rise to a large number of contour irregularities, such as rippling, waviness, and depressions in the skin. It wasn't unusual to suction large amounts of fat, sometimes with untoward results. Among other problems, many patients lost significant amounts of blood and body fluids as the cannula was swept around under their skin. Blood transfusions were often necessary. Patients also experienced substantial postoperative bruising and swelling. After the first few years of liposuction, it became apparent that there were limits to how much fat could be removed without threatening patients' health. Surgeons studied the outcome of hundreds of cases and designated a uniformly safe limit of about four and a half pounds of fat. This is substantially below the amount where complications would start to be seen. Remember, in cosmetic surgery, we are not trying to push the limits of human physiology. We are trying to be uniformly safe.

There were still other problems to be resolved. Early liposuction techniques resulted in a rippling of the skin over the treated areas. To correct that situation, surgeons began using more than one incision in order to suction fat from different angles. This advance may seem paradoxical because it results in multiple scars, but the approach minimizes rippling. This fundamental change occurred in the late 1980s, around the same time that smaller cannulas (suctioning tubes) gained in popularity. These narrower cannulas require smaller incisions and allow the surgeon to vacuum fat with greater precision. This reduced the number and severity of contour deformities. Blood loss, bruising, soreness, and fatigue continued to be problematic, however.

The next revolution was "tumescent liposuction," which cuts blood loss dramatically. To perform tumescent (derived from the Latin word meaning "to swell") liposuction, the surgeon first injects an infiltrating solution containing epinephrine and a very dilute anesthetic into the fat. Epinephrine—the "fight-or-flight" chemical also known as adrenaline—constricts blood vessels in the fat and skin. As a result, blood loss from the average liposuction patient dropped from more than a pint to less than half a pint. Tumescent liposuction thus obviated the need for a blood transfusion and allowed surgeons to safely exceed the previous four and a half-pound limit of fat removal. Postoperative discomfort is lessened since the anesthetic remains in the tissues for many hours after surgery. As an added bonus, tumescent liposuction resulted in less bruising, less fatigue, and faster resolution of swelling after the procedure. Liposuction continues to improve, but the tumescent technique is pretty much the standard used today.

How many people have had liposuction in the United States?

Millions have undergone this procedure since 1983. One survey of plastic surgeons found there were 51,072 liposuction procedures performed in 1994 alone—44,433 (87 percent) on women, and 6,639 (13 percent) on men. Almost half of those liposuction patients were between ages thirty-five and fifty; more than one-third were between nineteen and thirty-four years of age.

Why is liposuction the number-one cosmetic surgical procedure?

There are several explanations. First, liposuction happens to be a very effective method of removing stubborn deposits of fat, and the results are potentially permanent. Candidates for liposuction span all age groups from the late teens to the seventies. A majority of people gain weight as they get older. Aging baby boomers are discovering that it is increasingly difficult to lose that weight because their metabolism slows down. Even people who appear thin in clothing can have hidden fat in their thighs, belly, or neck that cannot be masked by a bathing suit.

Another reason for liposuction's popularity is that it can be performed on a wide variety of body parts, including the neck region to remove jowls and double chins, the upper arms, the male breasts, the abdomen, hips, lower buttock region, outer and inner thighs, lower back ("love handles"), knees, calves, and even ankles. There is a growing trend of having multiple body parts suctioned in one operation. Liposuction is an integral part of many face-lifts and other facial rejuvenation procedures.

Are there any parts of the body that should not be subjected to liposuction?

Most areas of the body can be suctioned, but some body parts are more "forgiving" than others. For example, it is hard to get a bad result on the hips but easy to be left with hanging skin on the inner thighs, which are very unforgiving. The abdomen and outer thighs are somewhat more forgiving. Jowls and double chins are relatively easy to correct with liposuction. Perhaps the least forgiving area is the buttock region, which is prone to dimpling and other contour deformities after liposuction unless the procedure is done very judiciously.

Is liposuction an alternative to weight-loss programs?

Absolutely not. Liposuction is neither an antidote for obesity nor a substitute for diet and exercise. Indeed, liposuction is best suited to remove isolated fat deposits that do not readily respond to conventional weight-loss efforts. Plastic surgeons prefer their liposuction patients to be within fifteen percent of their of ideal weight. Even people who have achieved their ideal weight can still exhibit "saddle bags" and other stubborn pockets of fat.

Excess fat deposits are a throwback to when our ancestors lived in caves. To help these early humans survive, fat was "programmed" through evolution to fuel the body at different rates depending on where it was located on the body. The last fat rations available to females are located primarily in the thighs and hips; in males, it is the abdomen. These emergency fat stores provided a survival advantage to cave dwellers, who sometimes were forced to go two or three months without food. In our era of bounty, you might starve yourself to get rid of all your "survival" fat. With liposuction, slimming down to an unhealthy weight can be avoided.

Can I have liposuction if I am obese?

Obese people should lose weight before they approach a plastic surgeon about liposuction. Why pay a consultation fee when the surgeon is probably going to turn you down or refer you to a weight-loss program, anyway? The problem with doing liposuction on obese people is knowing where to stop. Vacuuming large amounts of fat is unsafe.

How big are the cannulas?

Cannulas come in a variety of diameters and lengths to accommodate different body parts. The smallest ones are used on the face and neck; they range in diameter from 1½ to 3 millimeters and are 10 to 20 centimeters long. Cannulas used on the arms, legs, and torso are 3 to 6 millimeters in diameter and 10 to 40 centimeters long. All cannulas have one to three holes near the tip to let in fat that has been broken up.

Are there any medical conditions that would eliminate me as a liposuction candidate?

As with most cosmetic procedures, you should be in generally good health for liposuction. You should certainly avoid liposuction if you have a chronic medical condition, especially heart disease or kidney disease.

Simply telling your cosmetic surgeon that you are healthy isn't enough. During a preoperative consultation, your surgeon should examine you thoroughly, paying special attention to the fat and skin on areas you want treated. If your belly is to be suctioned, your surgeon should carefully examine your abdomen for hernias and scars. If you have a hernia your surgeon doesn't know about, it could be punctured during liposuction, especially with the new, smaller cannulas. If your neck is to be suctioned, that area should be examined to rule out any masses, cysts, or aneurysms.

If a surgeon agrees to perform liposuction before thoroughly examining you, you should worry about that doctor's competence. Conversely, if a plastic surgeon refuses to do liposuction for a medical reason, you could be putting your health or even your life at risk if you shop around for a surgeon willing to do the procedure. If you look hard enough, you will eventually find an unethical doctor who cares more about your money than your health.

What kind of anesthesia is used?

Tumescent liposuction, which is usually done on an outpatient basis, can be performed under local anesthesia with intravenous sedation, epidural anesthesia (a spinal block that numbs the lower half of the body), or general anesthesia. The choice of anesthesia depends on which parts of the body are being suctioned as well as the patient's desires and apprehensions. The operating room's capabilities also come into play. Generally, only small areas can be suctioned under local anesthesia with sedation. Only areas below the belly button can be suctioned under epidural anesthesia.

How is tumescent liposuction performed?

Prior to the procedure, you will be asked to stand naked as your surgeon uses a special marker to draw a topographic map of the fat on your body. (Body mapping is common in many cosmetic procedures.) The thickest fat layers are designated by the highest number of concentric circles. Mapping is important because your fat shifts and sinks into your body when you are laying down. Without the topographic lines, it would be difficult for the surgeon to know how much fat to suction from various regions.

At the conclusion of the mapping phase, you remain standing naked in the operating room as the surgeon or nurse paints your entire body with warmed orange betadine, a liquid disinfectant. The painting ritual is unique in cosmetic surgery and necessary because liposuction involves the front and back of your body. For example, if the doctor needs to suction both your abdomen and love handles, and betadine was applied while you were lying down, any unpainted areas would contaminate the operative field and put you at great risk of infection. Standing naked in the operating room is embarrassing, but the surgical staff is trained to maintain your dignity and complete the disinfecting task as quickly as possible, usually in a few minutes.

Once you are positioned on the operating table, an intravenous line is put in your arm so you can receive medications and fluids necessary to ward off dehydration. You will also be hooked to monitors that keep track of your vital signs. You will then be placed under general anesthesia or sedation, or receive an epidural catheter through which an anesthetic will flow into the area around your spinal cord.

The surgeon begins the operation by making a series of small incisions in appropriate locations on your body. The incisions, which were up to several inches long at the beginning of the liposuction era, are now less than one-quarter inch in length. Whenever possible, they are placed in natural skin creases, such as the bottom of the buttocks or the belly button. If the flanks are being suctioned, the surgeon has no choice but to make incisions out in the open, although there is enough leeway to be able to place the incisions so they can be hidden under a bathing suit.

Several liters of the epinephrine-anesthetic solution are then injected through the incisions. The solution causes your skin to bloat. After about eight minutes, your skin will turn from pink to white, meaning the epinephrine has taken effect. The surgeon can now insert cannulas through the same incisions and extract the fat into a specialized container that continuously measures the volume of tissue being removed. The surgeon judges the amount of fat removal by observing the ongoing result, by pinching the remaining fat and skin, and by comparing to the opposite side. Once fat removal is complete, the incisions are sutured closed and dressed.

You will have a restrictive garment placed on you while still in the operating room. For two weeks, this garment must be worn twenty-three hours a day. (There is an opening at the crotch for going to the bathroom.) For the next four weeks after that, you will wear a more casual garment sixteen to eighteen hours a day. Some patients take it off only to sleep; others prefer to take it off during work. The purpose of this tight-fitting girdle is to minimize the collection of fluid under your skin and to compress the holes created by the cannula. If you fail to wear the garment as recommended, your risk of contour irregularities increases.

Stitches are removed in about a week.

What will I see, feel, and hear if I am awake during liposuction?

A cannula moving around beneath your skin and yellowish fat flowing through tubing are not pretty sights, so a screen is usually placed blocking your view of the action. Even a curious, nonsqueamish patient ought not watch her own liposuction. You may feel some degree of discomfort as the area is anesthetized, but you should feel none as the fat is vacuumed out of your body. If the procedure is done correctly, there is remarkably little pain immediately after the operation.

The only sounds you will hear are the voices of your surgical team, the blaring of music on the radio, and the hum of the liposuction equipment. Some machines are louder than others, with the more expensive machines being the quietest.

How does the surgeon know how much fat to remove?

That is a judgment call based on the surgeon's experience. As mentioned earlier, the generally accepted limit is about four and a half pounds of fat, although some surgeons believe that with the tumescent technique, it is safe to remove more.

How long does liposuction take?

The length of the procedure depends on how many body parts are being suctioned. Thighs take about an hour, as does the abdomen. Knees can be suctioned in about half an hour; jowls and double chins take about forty-five minutes.

What happens to all those liters of epinephrine-anesthetic solution that were injected into my body?

The fluid is absorbed and eliminated through your urine. The drugs, which are kept to safe amounts, are metabolized, or destroyed, by your body.

What happens to all the fat that was suctioned out of my body?

It is processed as medical waste and disposed of along with blood, needles, and used gauze. Suctioned fat is not sent to a pathologist because it is considered normal tissue.

Can liposuction eliminate cellulite?

No. There have been claims by different physicians that various techniques, such as extremely superficial liposuction, can help. However, these techniques are not generally accepted procedures, and their value is in doubt.

Despite the heavily advertised anticellulite creams and exercise equipment, it is important to realize that cellulite is not a real entity. It is the visible manifestation of fibrous bands that tether your skin to underlying muscle. Cellulite appears as the skin loses elasticity, which sometimes occurs in the teens. For many people, cellulite rears its head during their twenties and worsens with each decade. Even if the tethers are cut, they will reattach themselves by virtue of scar tissue. A thigh-lift (see Chapter Fourteen) is the only procedure that can have an impact on cellulite because it removes excess skin and tightens remaining skin. In actuality, cellulite is not being reduced, it is just being stretched out by the thigh-lift.

What complications are possible with liposuction?

There are two categories of complications: aesthetic and medical. The most common aesthetic complications are contour irregularities, which can manifest in rippling, waviness, or dimpling of the skin over the suctioned areas. These irregularities can make your skin look worse than it did before liposuction, like very bad cellulite. Other potential problems are having too much fat left behind or too much taken away. There also could be asymmetry, especially visible in the inner thighs.

Ten to 20 percent of liposuction patients experience a contour irregularity severe enough to require a touchup procedure. Most surgeons do not charge for touchups, and most can be done under local anesthesia, but there probably will be another operating-room fee and, if necessary, an anesthesiologist's bill. You should wait until the swelling has gone down—at least three months after surgery before considering a touchup.

Whether you will need or want a touchup depends largely on the quality of your skin and your lifestyle. If a patient is in her teens, twenties, or thirties and has extremely tight skin, her likelihood of a contour irregularity is extremely low. By contrast, a forty-five-year-old with excess fat, sagging skin, and cellulite has a very high likelihood of contour irregularities after liposuction. These distortions are virtually impossible to fix unless, for example, you are willing to undergo a thigh lift—a major undertaking.

To be sure, there are many patients who don't care if their results are less than perfect. One woman in her mid-sixties had her protruding abdomen suctioned so she would look better in a one-piece bathing suit. Even though she was left with an unattractive, wavy belly, it was relatively flat—an acceptable tradeoff, in her eyes. Before surgery, she had been told of the very high likelihood of this result; her expectations were realistic. She was so happy with her new body that she came back to have her neck suctioned.

Aside from aesthetic complications, there are a number of potentially serious and even life-threatening medical complications that can result from liposuction. These include blood clots, dehydration, and perforating internal organs—with possibly fatal results. Most plastic surgeons decline to do lower body liposuction on people who have had blood clots in their legs. People with varicose veins are usually turned down, as well.

Has anyone ever died from liposuction?

Yes. Of the approximately five million liposuction cases done since 1983, there have been about fifteen reported deaths. Virtually every internal organ has been punctured by a liposuction cannula, including the heart, liver, and spleen. Catastrophic complications such as these are exceedingly rare, but they can happen. This underscores the importance of finding a competent, experienced surgeon who understands the fundamentals of surgery, anatomy, and physiology, and selects liposuction patients with the utmost care.

What will I look like after liposuction?

Your body will be black and blue for up to three weeks following liposuction. The swelling will last for six weeks with tumescent techniques and two to three months after nontumescent liposuction. Most patients take three or four days off work if they had liposuction on their torso or limbs. If liposuction was confined to the neck or face, you'll probably need to hide for about ten days to allow the bruises to fade. In most cases, 70 percent of the swelling is gone by three weeks, and 90 percent has disappeared by six weeks after the operation. Recent studies have found residual swelling and changes in the fat for many months following surgery.

What will the scars look like?

Over the next twelve months, your scars will fade significantly. They will be no bigger than the scar left behind after having a mole removed.

What does liposuction cost?

There is a lot of variability among surgeons' fee structures. Some charge about $2,500 for the first area (both outer thighs qualifying as a single area) plus $1,000 for each additional area. Other surgeons have standard fees for each area.

Anesthesiologists typically charge $500 for one area and $50 for each subsequent area. An outpatient facility costs in the $700 range for the first area plus $50 to $100 for each subsequent area. Hospital-based operating rooms are more expensive. Restrictive garments generally cost the patient $35 to $100, depending on their size and manufacturer; often, the surgeon's fee includes the cost of one or two garments.

How long after the procedure can I have sex?

You can usually have gentle sex one week after liposuction. Restrictive garments are designed so you need not take it off to have sex or go to the bathroom.

When can I take a shower?

You may shower the day after surgery. Your restrictive garment is designed to be worn in the shower, drying like a bathing suit.

When can I start exercising again?

You should avoid exercising for three weeks after liposuction. After that, you may gradually get back into your exercise routine. Contact sports should not be played for six weeks following surgery.

Are the results of liposuction permanent?

If you take in no more calories each day than you need to maintain your current weight, the results of your liposuction should be permanent.

Will I lose weight as a result of liposuction?

You will drop several pounds, but the scale should not be a motivating factor for having this procedure. The purpose of liposuction is to give your body a more attractive silhouette, not to help you lose weight.

What happens if I gain weight after liposuction?

You will gain weight everywhere on your body, but not as much in the suctioned areas. The reason: There are fewer fat cells in the places that were suctioned. Like muscle cells, fat cells can grow larger but do not increase in number after about age twelve.

How many inches can I expect to lose after liposuction?

That varies widely, and most surgeons do not take before and after measurements of their liposuction patients. A better measure of the procedure's success is whether you look better in your clothes. Most people need to buy a slightly smaller size or find they are more comfortable wearing their existing wardrobe.

What is ultrasound-assisted liposuction?

Ultrasound-assisted liposuction (UAL) is the newest innovation to sweep the cosmetic surgery world. With traditional liposuction, a surgeon mechanically breaks up fat with a cannula. With UAL, ultrasonic waves emulsify the fat before it is vacuumed away. This new system has been used in Italy for about ten years and has been used by a handful of plastic surgeons in the United States working closely with the FDA to establish safety standards. In January 1997, a consortium of plastic surgery societies began an ambitious program to train the nation's plastic surgeons in the technique. Plastic surgeons now are beginning to perform UAL procedures across the country.

UAL holds great promise because it causes less bleeding

than traditional liposuction and is more effective in areas of fibrous fat, such as the male breasts, upper abdomen, and the back. The risks include all of the risks of liposuction plus seromas (fluid collections) under the skin and burns to the skin. UAL takes more time then traditional liposuction and may require the placement of drains in the skin for a few days.

Researchers are also investigating whether UAL's aesthetic results are better than those achieved with tumescent liposuction. Many plastic surgeons do not think there is much difference, except in the aforementioned areas of fibrous fat. However, ultrasound-assisted liposuction is new and high-tech, so expect the press to glamorize it and the public to demand it. It is likely that UAL will be significantly more expensive than standard liposuction. UAL equipment costs $40,000, compared with about $3,000 for a traditional liposuction machine.

❖ 14 ❖

BODY CONTOURING

Tummy Tuck, Thigh-Lift, Buttock-Lift

What is "body contouring?"

"Body contouring" is an umbrella term for a variety of surgical procedures that reshape the body by removing or manipulating fat, skin, and muscle. Liposuction (see Chapter Thirteen) is one form of body contouring that focuses solely on fat removal through small tubes. This chapter throws a spotlight on the more aggressive body-contouring operations being performed by plastic surgeons: the tummy tuck, the thigh-lift, and the buttock-lift.

How common are these procedures?

In 1994, the 16,829 tummy tucks done in this country accounted for just over 4 percent of all cosmetic surgical procedures. The thigh-lift and buttock-lift were performed even less frequently, accounting for 0.3 percent (1,098 procedures) and less than 0.1 percent (314 procedures), respectively, according to the American Society of Plastic and Reconstructive Surgeons. Considering that there are about 4,000 plastic surgeons in the United States, that means only one in four did just one thigh-lift that year.

There are good reasons why these operations are not more popular. They leave enormous scars. They have a relatively high rate of complications, such as infections, blood loss, and blood clots. People undergoing these procedures must be able to take three weeks off from work and other daily routines to recuperate. Body-contouring operations are also quite expensive.

The good news is that these operations can be extraordinarily effective in transforming extremely unattractive tummies, thighs, and buttocks into sources of pride.

Who is the typical candidate for a tummy tuck?

Most tummy-tuck patients are women who have given birth to one or more children. The belly protrudes not necessarily because it is covered by too much fat, but because the two abdominal (rectus) muscles have been overstretched. The rectus muscles drift apart to make way for the burgeoning uterus, much like a man's suspenders drift to either side to accommodate a beer belly. After the baby is born, the rectus muscles never fully return to their pre-pregnancy positions—unless you are Jane Fonda. The looseness this creates in the abdominal wall allows the intestines and other abdominal organs to push the abdominal skin forward. No amount of exercise can completely reverse this condition.

How can a tummy tuck help?

A tummy tuck, or abdominoplasty, can flatten the protruding belly by removing excess skin and fat and, if necessary, by sewing the rectus muscles together to create an "inner girdle."

Can an obese person have a tummy tuck?

No. Most plastic surgeons select patients for this procedure who are no more than 15 percent over their ideal body weight. If you weigh more than that, you will probably be referred to a weight-loss program before being reconsidered for this surgery.

Morbidly obese individuals may be candidates for a panniculectomy, a surgical procedure that removes excess skin that often results from significant weight loss. A panniculectomy is appropriate where three to six inches of excess skin is hanging off the abdomen. This procedure is done to facilitate personal hygiene and to assist in the weight-loss program.

How can I tell if I need a tummy tuck, or whether liposuction would suffice?

If your abdominal skin hangs loose and has numerous stretch marks, liposuction is generally ill-advised because it will result in more loose skin and has no impact on stretch marks. Another indication for a tummy tuck would be if you have very little fat but your stomach bulges anyway. In cases where there is both excess fat and a weakened abdominal wall, liposuction can be performed along the flanks and sides of the abdomen just prior to the abdominoplasty. Liposuction should not be performed on the middle of the belly, however, because it would result in too much trauma to the abdominal skin when followed by a tummy tuck.

What kind of anesthesia is used for the tummy tuck?

Abdominoplasty is almost always performed while the patient is under general anesthesia.

Where do the incisions go?

There are three types of tummy tuck incisions that are popular. The classic W-shaped incision begins at either hipbone and descends diagonally to just above the pubic hairline.

If the patient has had a C-section, the tummy-tuck incision can be superimposed on the C-section incision and extended upward to the hipbones, creating a half-circle.

Recently, some plastic surgeons have started doing what's known as the "high lateral tension abdominoplasty" through an incision across the lower belly that angles sharply upward at the sides, along the lines of a French-cut bathing suit. This approach places more tension on the side portions of the incision rather than the middle, allegedly improving the appearance of the scar.

Regardless of the shape and position of the primary incision, a secondary incision around the belly button is also needed so it can be freed up from surrounding skin.

A new twist to the tummy tuck is the endoscopic abdominoplasty. Through tiny, remote incisions in the pubic hair and belly button, the muscles of the belly are tightened. Liposuction can also be performed, but no skin is removed, so this is appropriate only for a minority of patients.

What happens after the incisions are made?

In a traditional tummy tuck, the skin over the belly is separated from underlying tissue and lifted all the way to the bottom of the ribcage. The belly button is lifted, too, but remains attached to underlying tissue. The surgeon may, if necessary, gently cut away a limited amount of excess fat from the upper portion of the skin flap. If the rectus muscles are apart, they are brought together and sutured down the middle to create the inner-girdle effect. Next, all the skin from the level of the belly button to the pubic hairline is removed. The remaining skin is pulled down very tightly. The surgeon cuts a hole in the appropriate location on the skin flap for the belly button. The edges of skin are sewn together, and stitches are placed around the belly button to hold it in place on its new skin. Several temporary drains are placed in the operative area to prevent fluid buildup. The drains look like little grenades about the size of tennis balls that suck out the fluid. This helps the skin heal down to the underlying tissue. You will be instructed on how to empty the grenades as they fill up and record how much fluid they collected until they are removed one to four days after surgery.

Will my belly button look any different after the operation?

The position of your belly button will not change, but its appearance probably will. There are various techniques to try to make an aesthetically pleasing belly button, and it usually ends up looking very normal.

How will I feel when I wake up from surgery?

Once the operation is over, there will be a great feeling of tightness and some degree of muscle spasms in your abdomen. There will also be a moderate amount of abdominal pain, which can be controlled through medication. You will be mostly bedridden except to use the bathroom and eat for the first forty-eight hours. You must lie on your back in a jackknife position, with your head and feet elevated about 15 degrees. Before leaving home for surgery, get your bed ready by placing about four inches of books under the foot of your mattress. You'll also need three pillows, one to support your upper back and two to support your head.

Where are abdominoplasties performed?

The tummy tuck can be performed in an outpatient setting only if the abdominal muscles do not need repair. However, if your abdominal muscles are to be sewn together, the tummy tuck becomes a four-hour operation that should be done on an inpatient basis. Remaining hospitalized for at least one night is important because 25 to 30 percent of people become nauseated after general anesthesia. That nausea must be controlled because if you vomit within the first day after surgery, it can destroy the muscle repair or trigger bleeding that could require emergency surgery.

What risk factors are associated with a tummy tuck?

All the skin lifting and pulling involved in this operation, as well as fat removal, combine to markedly decrease blood flow to the abdominal skin. As a result, 1 or 2 percent of patients suffer some degree of abdominal skin loss, which in extreme cases requires a skin graft. There have been cases where all the skin across the abdomen died as a result of the operation. For this reason, many plastic surgeons refuse to perform tummy tucks or any skin-lifting procedures on smokers, diabetics, and people with small blood-vessel diseases such as rheumatoid arthritis, because of their preexisting diminished blood flow in the skin.

Another potentially devastating complication is the formation of blood clots in the legs. A few tummy-tuck patients have actually died from pulmonary embolisms, or blood clots that travel from the legs to the lungs, and a handful have suffered heart attacks. To reduce these risks, tummy-tuck patients may be given a blood-thinning drug such as heparin just prior to surgery. Wearing compression boots on the legs during surgery also helps prevent clots.

About 5 percent of tummy-tuck patients have postoperative bleeding between the abdominal skin and underlying muscles, which requires another trip to the operating room. Postoperative bleeding occurs more frequently with the tummy tuck than with any other procedure in plastic surgery. The main symptoms are rapid swelling, bleeding, and severe abdominal pain. The chance of bleeding can often be minimized by plenty of bed rest and inactivity for at least two days after the operation.

Another risk is the collection of fluid under the abdominal skin, although the temporary drains under the skin flap prevent fluid buildup in the vast majority of cases.

Clearly, while the tummy tuck offers wonderful aesthetic benefits, there are some profound risks associated with this procedure. Patients must be very serious in deciding to have this operation and willing to accept all the risks.

Are there any medical conditions that would disqualify me from having a tummy tuck?
Generally speaking, the tummy tuck is only for people in good health. Because of the potential for serious com-

plications, plastic surgeons are extra cautious in selecting patients for this procedure. Having high blood pressure is not a problem as long as it is effectively treated with medication.

What is the cost of this procedure?

Plastic surgeons generally charge between $4,000 and $6,000 for a tummy tuck; the anesthesiologist's fee is $1,500 or more. If you are to be hospitalized after surgery, expect to pay another $3,000 to $5,000 or so for the operating room and overnight stay.

Historically, tummy-tuck expenses have been covered in part or in full by medical insurance, although coverage is quickly becoming less likely owing to cost-containment measures throughout the industry. Insurance may cover the operation if your abdominal muscles are overstretched enough to cause such symptoms as chronic back pain, posture problems, or abdominal discomfort.

Will I need a blood transfusion during surgery?

Thanks to modern surgical techniques, tummy tucks rarely result in enough blood loss to warrant a transfusion.

Can abdominoplasty get rid of stretch marks and old scars?

Yes, depending on their location. All abdominal stretch marks and old scars beneath the level of your belly button will be gone forever after the operation. So will any hair that grew on your lower belly.

How much swelling and bruising will I experience after surgery?

You will experience a tremendous amount of swelling but not too much bruising as all the cut blood vessels are cauterized during a tummy tuck. Much of the swelling will be gone three weeks after surgery, and the rest will disappear by about three months.

Will I need to wear a girdle during the recovery period?

Usually the patient wears an abdominal binder garment twenty-four hours a day for the first two weeks after surgery and sixteen to eighteen hours a day for the next four weeks. Wearing the garment decreases fluid collections and molds the skin. Most patients feel better with the binder on and are reluctant to give it up when it is no longer needed.

Will there be much pain?

Yes, not so much when you are lying still, but when you move about. Your abdominal muscles tend to spasm when they are moved. Most patients need narcotic painkillers for about a week after a tummy tuck, longer than any other cosmetic procedure. Also, because so much skin was removed, most patients cannot stand fully erect for at least a week. It takes that long for the abdominal skin to stretch into its new position.

When can I shower?

You can shower one day after your drains are removed—two to five days after surgery.

How soon can I have sex?

You should wait at least two weeks after your tummy tuck before engaging in sexual activity, as long as it is gentle. By three weeks, you may fully resume your normal sexual relations.

When do the stitches come out?

Superficial stitches will be removed by the seventh day after surgery. A second, deeper layer of stitches will stay in many months before they dissolve.

Will I have reduced sensation on my abdomen?

This always happens where skin has been lifted during surgery. It generally takes three months for sensation to return to normal.

What will the scars look like?

Unlike facial cosmetic surgery where the incisions are very well hidden, there is no way to hide the tummy tuck scar. It is more than a foot long. Ninety-five percent of these scars remain fairly thin, less than one-quarter-inch wide, and turn white after six to twelve months. In 5 percent of patients, however, the scar winds up as an unsightly red, wide line. The belly button scar is usually far less noticeable.

Fortunately, the primary scar gets hidden under all types of underwear and most one- and two-piece bathing suits, as long as it is not a thong bikini. In some cases, the surgeon can alter the incision to accommodate a particular type of bathing suit you wish to wear.

Is there anything I can do to make the scar less obvious?

Not really. If your scar becomes red, you can try a silicone sheet that may help the scar mature a little faster. No one knows why this works, but it is thought to heat up the skin by several degrees, thereby increasing the rate of natural scar-tissue breakdown. Sometimes, steroids are injected into the scars to speed their maturation.

How long after surgery can I start exercising my abdominal muscles?

You should refrain from doing any exercises that challenge your abdominal muscles for two or three months after surgery.

When can I ride a stationary bike or do other aerobic exercises that don't work the abdominal muscles directly?

You should do no exercise at all for the first three weeks after surgery. Over the following three weeks, you can start walking and doing very mild exercises, gradually building up to your regular aerobic exercise routine six weeks after surgery.

Will my waist size be smaller after abdominoplasty?
Yes, you will lose several inches from your waistline.

How many dress sizes can I expect to drop after all the swelling goes down?
Most women drop at least one dress size after a tummy tuck.

Will I weigh less after surgery?
You will probably lose two to four pounds from the skin and fat that were removed combined with a starvation diet around the time of surgery.

How long will my tummy tuck last?
The results of this operation should be permanent. If you gain weight or become pregnant, however, you will have a recurrence of protruding abdomen, although to a lesser extent than before your tummy tuck.

What is the satisfaction rate among abdominoplasty patients?
Quite high. It is important to realize that the tummy tuck is a compromise operation: You must be willing to accept health risks, a long recovery period, considerable pain, and substantial scarring in exchange for a flat, tight tummy.

Can a tummy tuck be combined with a thigh-lift in one operation?
No. Both are major, lengthy procedures. It would be too risky to attempt both in one operation.

What is a thigh-lift?
The thigh-lift is a procedure to tighten sagging skin on the inner thighs, outer thighs, or both. The most popular

version is the inner thigh-lift because skin on the inner thigh is more prone to sagging than outer-thigh skin.

What kinds of people have thigh-lifts?

People who undergo this procedure are highly motivated. They have very unattractive thighs and are almost disgraced by them. They have done all the thigh-reduction exercises to no avail. They cannot wear bathing suits or shorts and are at their wits end.

How is the thigh-lift performed?

An incision is made in the groin crease and continues around the inside of the thigh to the buttock crease. If both inner and outer thighs are being lifted, the incision is circumferential. The skin is lifted off underlying tissue, and excess skin is removed. The remaining skin is pulled up and attached by sutures to the deep connective tissue of the thigh in the area of the groin to anchor it in its new position. Temporary drains are put in, and the incisions are closed.

How long does this procedure take?

The thigh-lift is a long, complicated undertaking that lasts anywhere from four to eight hours. Significant incisions are made, and the patient must be turned several times during the operation. Thigh-lifts are always done under general anesthesia and usually require a hospital stay of one to two nights.

What risks are associated with the thigh-lift?

The medical risks are the same as the those of the tummy tuck—including postoperative bleeding and blood clots—but are more likely to occur.

Can I combine liposuction with a thigh-lift?

Liposuction (see Chapter Thirteen) can be done very cautiously and very judiciously during the thigh-lift operation. It is far better to have liposuction of your thighs three to six months prior to your thigh-lift. In fact, thinning the fat beforehand makes the thigh-lift an immensely easier procedure with smoother, better-looking results and a lower complication rate. Liposuction also can be done after a thigh-lift, although it could cause a recurrence of drooping skin.

What does a thigh-lift cost?

The thigh-lift is one of the costliest procedures in cosmetic surgery. The surgeon's fee alone is typically more than $6,000. The anesthesiologist charges $1,500 or more. The operating room and hospitalization costs can exceed $5,000.

What is the recovery period like?

You will be confined to bed for the first day after surgery and may move about the second day with assistance. You can stand or lie down but you may not sit for several weeks after your thigh-lift or you might reopen your incisions. You will have the same physical activity restrictions as tummy-tuck patients, and you should refrain from sex for at least three weeks. You will need to wear compression boots or take heparin to reduce the chance of blood clots in your legs for several days after surgery.

How long will it take until I am completely healed?

By two months after your thigh-lift, you will be ready to jog.

Are most patients happy with the results of this surgery?

Yes. Despite all its complexity and potential complications, the thigh-lift is a very effective way of transforming unattractive thighs into nice-looking thighs that patients are eager to show off. Because of the scars, however, you must be careful in choosing bathing suits, but you can wear short shorts without a problem.

Is the buttock-lift as successful as the thigh-lift?

No. The buttock is the great unsolved area of cosmetic surgery. Surgical procedures to reduce the buttock's size, tighten drooping skin, and give the rear end a more attractive contour are not yet perfected. The procedures that are available have so many drawbacks that most people don't want to go through them. The best technique leaves big scars, and results are variable and not as predictable as they are with the thigh-lift and tummy tuck.

Another reason the buttock-lift is so unpopular is because patients cannot sit down for three weeks after surgery.

How is a buttock lift performed?

An incision is made along the crease below the buttocks, and the skin is lifted. Excess skin and fat are removed, and the skin is sewn down into its new position.

Can a buttock-lift get rid of cellulite?

The operation can make the rear end look a little tighter, but it probably will not improve the fine depressions and rippling on the buttock skin. Also, buttock skin can begin to sag again a few years after the procedure. Even slight sagging will reveal any imperfections in the skin or underlying tissue layers.

❖ 15 ❖

TEEN SCENE

Cosmetic Surgery on Children and Teenagers

What are the top cosmetic procedures performed on young people?

Nose reshaping, or rhinoplasty (see Chapter Nine), is by far the most popular cosmetic surgery among the eighteen and younger set. More than 4,300 American teenagers had rhinoplasty in 1994, according to the most recent data from the American Society of Plastic and Reconstructive Surgeons. Next is otoplasty, or ear-setback surgery. Slightly more than half of all otoplasties performed in this country are done on patients aged eighteen and younger. Male breast reduction to correct a condition known as gynecomastia ranks third. Other cosmetic procedures done on young people include chin augmentation (see Chapter Five), breast enlargement (see Chapter Ten), breast reduction (see Chapter Twelve), and dermabrasion (see Chapter Six).

What is the best age for children to have cosmetic surgery?

That decision depends on a variety of factors, including which operation is being considered, who your surgeon is, the parents' feelings, and the child's desire and level of emotional and physical maturity. For rhinoplasty, it is best to wait until the nose bones have stopped growing. This is generally when the child's facial height has reached that of the parent's. Fourteen is the youngest generally accepted age for both rhinoplasty and chin augmentation, although some youngsters may be prepared physically and emotionally at a younger age. At fourteen years, however, the basic length and shape of the chin and nose are established. There are situations—such as after a fracture or if the child has a severe congenital deformity—where the surgery can be done earlier in life.

Ear setback can be performed on children as young as five, when 90 percent of ear growth is complete.

If gynecomastia is extreme, male breast reduction can be performed on someone as young as fourteen. Plastic surgeons usually prefer to wait until the patient is in his late teens or early twenties, however, because gynecomastia is temporary in the vast majority of cases.

Breast enlargement should not be performed on girls under age seventeen or eighteen, when sexual maturity is complete. The rule of thumb for breast reduction is to wait at least one year after the emergence of secondary sex characteristics, although if it is done very early, it may have to be repeated after additional breast growth has occurred.

Does cosmetic surgery have a more dramatic impact on children compared with adults?

This is undeniably the case. Personality is malleable in children, adolescents, and teenagers. Traits such as introversion can develop from a physical feature that is perceived as ugly or abnormal. Being called "Dumbo" because his ears stick out or "Pinocchio" if her nose is too big can crush a youngster's sense of self-esteem before it has a chance to solidify.

Physical appearance and peer acceptance are never more important than they are during school years. Just clock how many hours teenagers spend in front of the mirror. Teens' obsession over their looks has been fortified by research showing that attractive girls and boys tend to have more friends than unattractive kids and may actually be treated better by their teachers. One fourteen-year-old girl who received rhinoplasty, chin augmentation, and acne medication simultaneously experienced a complete personality transformation within two months after surgery. Today she smiles more, talks more, and can look at herself in the mirror with admiration instead of disgust. Similarly, a thirty-one-year-old woman who had rhinoplasty at age sixteen says that her new nose literally transformed her from a shy, self-conscious teenager to a confident, outgoing one. The primary reason otoplasty is done on five-year-olds is to spare them the taunting that would otherwise ensue when they enter school.

With their personalities still in the larval stage, youngsters adapt easily to changes in their appearance—even dramatic changes. By contrast, adults, whose personality and self-image are ingrained, are usually happiest with subtle changes that make them look like a younger version of themselves.

If I encourage my child to have cosmetic surgery, am I sending the message that one's appearance means more than one's character and intelligence?

Of course not. The goal of cosmetic surgery, particularly among young people, is to make people look "normal" so they will feel more comfortable with themselves. Indeed, getting teased or feeling self-conscious about a physical feature might interfere with a young person's character development and ability to learn.

On the other hand, no parent should drag their child kicking and screaming into a plastic surgeon's office. If a child over age ten or twelve is not bothered by a physical feature that you, the parent, perceive as problematic, there is no need to create self-consciousness where it did not exist before.

A more typical scenario would be an adolescent or teenager who dislikes an aspect of his or her appearance but doesn't realize that surgery can help. In these instances, you can delicately inform your son or daughter that there are procedures to reshape the nose or correct other problems, and you are open to discussion should he or she ever want to talk about it. Most plastic surgeons would be happy to put your child in touch with someone close to their age who has undergone cosmetic surgery.

Karen, a thirty-nine-year-old speech therapist, jokes that her mother decided when she was an infant that she would need rhinoplasty. "She was always conscious that I had my father's nose. She would say, 'Turn yourself this way so your nose won't look so big' whenever I had my picture taken," Karen remembers. "My brother had my father's nose, too, but it was less acceptable on a girl."

Karen doesn't know if the bump on her nose would have bothered her if her mother had never made an issue of it. She then recalled a classmate whose nose was bigger than hers but was nevertheless the most popular girl in school. "She was a cheerleader, class president, very self-assured," Karen says.

Karen, a mother of two preadolescent girls, is currently witnessing the emergence of her father's nose bump on her nine-year-old daughter, Julie. "In a few years, I think I would bring it around to conversation that I had had the surgery. I might say that I had Poppy's nose, too. It's a very nice nose, but it kind of looked big on my face, and that there is surgery available. I would tell her that if any time down the road she wants it, that it is a possibility," Karen says. "I guess I just want to open the door without giving her a complex. I wouldn't say what my mother said to me, but of course I might say something else stupid."

How can I keep my youngster's expectations of cosmetic surgery realistic?

Children don't really have expectations of cosmetic surgery until they reach twelve to fourteen years of age. Even then, they are not mature enough to fully understand all the nuances and implications of surgery. They simply want to get rid of a problem that makes other people tease them.

People aged fifteen and older have a more sophisticated understanding of their problem and are better able to articulate what troubles them: "My nose is too wide," or "I don't like this hook (or bump) on my nose." But they also tend to be on a quest for perfection. They may tear out magazine pictures of their favorite musicians, actors, actresses, or models and fantasize that surgery can make them just as beautiful. The parent and plastic surgeon must work together to convince these teens that such high expectations are unrealistic and can set them up for disappointment. Most fifteen-year-olds are mature enough to understand what cosmetic surgery can and cannot do. If there is any doubt about their understanding, the operation is best postponed until the teenager is older.

How do I know if my teenaged son or daughter is a good candidate for cosmetic surgery?

The teen must have a bona fide anatomical abnormality and be able to understand and accept the potential for postoperative complications. The surgeon must be convinced that the patient has enough emotional maturity not to go to pieces if something goes wrong. The teen should also be able to develop a rapport with the surgeon and demonstrate a willingness to follow the doctor's instructions. For example, by ignoring the advice against touching the area that was operated on until it is fully healed, the child could damage the stitches, cause bleeding, or introduce infection.

In one case, a surgeon canceled rhinoplasty on a fourteen-year-old girl an hour before the procedure was scheduled to begin. "I felt that she did not have a good grasp of what we could reasonably accomplish in the operating room,'' the doctor explains. ''She was mute and refused to talk about her feelings to me or her parents. She wouldn't even look me in the eye. I began to feel more and more uneasy.

''You've got to be in command of yourself in order to have a procedure like this,'' the surgeon continues. ''The patient has to be able to work with me and talk with me throughout the whole postoperative period. I have to know she won't be suicidal if it turns out that she needs more surgery.''

Do kids heal faster from cosmetic surgery than adults?

There can be some slight differences in healing rates, but children and healthy adults generally heal at a similar pace. Children do tend to make much more scar tissue than adults, and that is not to the youngsters' advantage. Fortunately, scars from the top two procedures—rhinoplasty and otoplasty—are hidden from view.

What causes protruding ears?

Ear protrusion is a developmental defect in which the ear cartilage fails to fold back toward the head properly. As a result the ears stick out. Ear protrusion is more of a problem for boys since they tend to wear their hair short. Girls can cover the defect with long hair. However, as they grow older, protruding ears may prevent them from wearing their hair short, pinning it back, or showing off earrings.

How does otoplasty correct this problem?

The surgeon makes a small incision behind the ear to access the cartilage. Several cuts are made in the cartilage and permanent stitches are placed in such a way as to tack the ear back into a normal position. In some instances, some ear cartilage is removed, as well. Once the permanent sutures are in place, the skin is sewn closed, and the ears bandaged. The bandages are worn for a week before the outside stitches are removed. After that, a sweatbandlike splint is worn day and night for about six weeks to keep the ears folded back. The child must refrain from all sports during this recovery period.

The surgery itself takes two to three hours. If the child wants the surgery and is cooperative, it can be done under local anesthesia with sedation. Otoplasty is usually done as an outpatient procedure.

What risks are associated with otoplasty?

As with all surgeries, there is a risk of infection, scarring, deformity of the ears, and a recurrence of the original deformity if the permanent stitches break within the first month after surgery. This happens to about 5 percent of patients. Parents must drill "Don't touch your ears!" into the child's head over and over throughout the healing process.

What does otoplasty cost?

The surgeon's fee generally ranges from $2,000 to $3,000. The patient's family is charged another $1,500 or so for the anesthesiologist and operating room. Medical insurance frequently covers otoplasty because ear protrusion is considered a developmental abnormality. Coverage will probably be less available in the future as managed care continues to grow.

Is male breast reduction covered by insurance?

In many cases, the answer is yes. Like protruding ears, gynecomastia is considered a developmental abnormality.

What causes gynecomastia?

Gynecomastia, a swelling of one or both breasts, usually stems from an imbalance of estrogen and testosterone in the blood. Sixty-four percent of adolescent males produce enough estrogen to develop slight breast swelling, which peaks around age fourteen. In the vast majority of adolescent cases, gynecomastia disappears spontaneously within two years. If breast swelling persists beyond age twenty or becomes too excessive to hide under clothing, breast-reduction surgery may be warranted. Before having surgery, the patient should be examined by an endocrinologist, an internist who specializes in the endocrine system, to rule out glandular diseases and tumors that can spur an overproduction of estrogen.

Many types of drugs, such as marijuana, can cause gynecomastia, as can heredity, liver disease (usually in older men), and certain birth defects, including Klinefelter's syndrome, a chromosomal abnormality that affects about one out of five hundred male babies. A significant number of men over age sixty-five develop gynecomastia, possibly because their testosterone level is dropping faster than their estrogen level, their use of various prescription drugs, or because of obesity.

In adolescents, sometimes waiting two years to see if breast swelling subsides can do more harm than good, psychologically speaking. Such was the case fourteen-year-old Danny whose breasts had grown to the size of a D cup. He was so mortified by his condition that he refused to go to school, wear a bathing suit or T-shirt, or participate in sports or social activities. After recovering from his operation, Danny's personality improved dramatically. He launched into a weight-training program, as advised by his surgeon, to build up his pectoral (chest) muscles. The exercises helped Danny develop a more masculine chest.

What is involved in male breast-reduction surgery?

The patient is given general anesthesia, or local anesthesia with sedation. An incision is made around the border of the areola, from the 3 o'clock to 9 o'clock positions. Working through the incision, the surgeon cuts away all the breast tissue between the skin and muscle. Liposuction (see Chapter Thirteen) is then used to remove excess fat from the area around the breasts. Drains are placed, and the incision is sewn closed and bandaged. The patient is given a tight-fitting vest to wear for the next six weeks. The drains are removed in three or four days. Stitches come out a week after surgery. The patient should refrain from upper-body exercise for at least six weeks.

Won't the stretched-out breast skin droop after surgery?

This is not usually a problem in young people, whose skin has plenty of elastin and conforms readily to the new chest contour. If the operation leaves excess skin, surgery can be performed later to remove it.

Will the scars be visible?

By placing the incision around the areola, the scar becomes very difficult to see once it matures. Scar maturation takes up to a year.

How much does male breast-reduction surgery cost?

The surgeon's fee ranges from about $4,500 to $5,500 for this three-hour procedure, which can be done on an inpatient or outpatient basis. The anesthesiologist's fee is in the neighborhood of $1,000, and the operating room charge is about $2,000 to $3,000, depending on whether it is hospital-based or office-based.

Is there anything I can tell my children that might help them avoid the need for a face-lift or other rejuvenation procedures later in life?

Using strong sunscreens (SPF 15 or higher) religiously is the most important thing youngsters can do to protect their skin from cancer and premature aging. You can say this until the cows come home, but children and teenagers feel immortal, and most couldn't care less about something that might happen thirty years down the road. It isn't until they reach their midtwenties that they begin to understand their mortality and vulnerability to ultraviolet light. Finally, your warning will start to make sense. Unfortunately, much of the damage is already done if your children had sustained multiple sunburns over the years.

Therefore, the role of the parent is to lay down the law and continually demand that sunscreens be used on a regular basis. Let your children see you apply sunscreen to your own skin. If you start when your kids are toddlers, there is a chance that your healthy habit will—if you'll pardon the pun—rub off on them.

❖ 16 ❖

TERRIFIC TEETH

Cosmetic Dentistry

What is cosmetic dentistry?

Cosmetic dentistry encompasses a range of procedures that enhance the teeth aesthetically without necessarily altering their function. In its simplest form, removing an old silver filling and replacing it with a tooth-colored one can be considered cosmetic dentistry. Orthodontics (braces) straighten the teeth, close gaps, and often improve function as well as aesthetics. Other popular cosmetic dental procedures include bleaching; bonding and porcelain veneers to whiten the teeth and even change their shape; "microabrasion," a technique to remove superficial stains from tooth enamel; and aesthetic recontouring, or reshaping the teeth with a specialized grinding stone.

How has cosmetic dentistry changed over the last ten years?

The field of cosmetic dentistry has exploded in many respects, ranging from biological research to materials and techniques to computer imaging and design to intraoral photography.

In the past, a dentist would need to draw pictures and use models to explain to patients how cosmetic dentistry can help them. Today, a dentist can photograph patients' teeth with a sophisticated camera and project these images on a fifteen- or twenty-inch video screen. The same images can be digitized, loaded into a computer, and manipulated with a mouse and keyboard to show how various cosmetic procedures might improve a patient's smile. The dentist can then print out "before" and "after" images to include in a treatment proposal to the patient. In the near future, dentists will have the technology to create many types of porcelain restorations at the chair side instead of making patients wait a day or more for dental labs to do the work.

As the cosmetic dentistry field continues to advance, it is attracting both patients and talent to the world of smile enhancement. The Madison, Wisconsin–based American Academy of Cosmetic Dentistry had a mere thirty members when it was formed in 1984. Today, more than three thousand dentists are on its membership roster.

How do I find a cosmetic dentist?

Any licensed dentist may legally perform cosmetic dentistry, although not all are experienced with every cosmetic procedure. Ask your dentist how comfortable he or she is with cosmetic dentistry and how much training and experience he or she has in the type of procedure you are interested in. Most dentists can provide composite fillings and dental bleaching. If your dentist does not do bonding and other more sophisticated procedures, ask for a referral to someone who does. Ideally, you want a dentist who has done your procedure hundreds of times. Other dental specialists, such as prosthodontists (dentists who focus on tooth-replacement procedures) and periodontists (dentists who specialize in gum disease) may have a special interest in cosmetic dentistry, as well. In addition to your dentist, referrals can come from friends and relatives who have had cosmetic dentistry and are happy with the results.

Membership in a cosmetic dentistry professional group does not necessarily guarantee competence as cosmetic dentistry is not at this writing a specialty that is recognized by the American Dental Association.

Are there any medical conditions that would rule someone out for cosmetic dentistry?

Medical problems are generally not an issue with most cosmetic dental procedures, which focus on the teeth and don't touch the gums. If, however, a procedure wounds or manipulates the gums or other soft tissue in the mouth, you could face healing problems if you have any systemic diseases such as diabetes, or if you are a heavy smoker. In addition, a thorough medical history should be obtained before undergoing any procedure requiring local anesthesia. There are some medications, such as Dilantin, which discolor gums and may negate restorative efforts.

Do dental plans ever cover cosmetic procedures?

If the procedure is purely cosmetic, don't expect it to be covered by your dental insurance. However, your insurance may provide full or partial reimbursement to replace old damaged fillings, crowns, or other restorations with modern, more aesthetically pleasing materials. Don't settle for a verbal approval of coverage from your insurer. Request a preapproval in writing before having your teeth worked on, if finances are a concern.

Is it possible to see beforehand what I'll look like after the procedure?

As with cosmetic plastic surgery, it is impossible to accurately predict the outcome of any cosmetic dental procedure. You can get an idea of what these procedures can accomplish by looking at "before" and "after" photographs of other patients who corrected problems similar to your own. Computer-enhanced images of your own teeth can also provide a clue, although the dentist must be careful not to enhance an image so much that it exceeds dentistry's limitations. Some dentists have interactive CD-ROMs that give patients information about what cosmetic dentistry can do and answer their questions.

Why do teeth become discolored?

There are several possible causes of tooth discoloration. One is your genetic program. The color of your teeth is determined to a large degree by the color of your dentin, the resilient material that constitutes the teeth's inner core. Just as eye, skin, and hair color vary from person to person, so does the color of dentin. Some people have whiter dentin while other people's dentin has a grayish, yellowish, or brownish hue. Dentin is covered by enamel, a relatively translucent material that allows the tooth's color to show through. The enamel's thickness, which also varies from person to person, influences its degree of translucency and thus how much dentin shows through.

As we get older, certain longtime habits, such as tobacco use and tea and coffee drinking, can result in discolored or stained teeth. In these cases, the discoloration may be uniform or manifest in brown patches or fine vertical lines. Another cause of tooth discoloration is from the antibiotic tetracycline, which can cause bluish-gray or brown lines or bands to form on teeth if taken while the teeth are forming in childhood.

How effective is tooth bleaching?

Discoloration stemming from tetracycline use are some of the hardest stains to get rid of through bleaching. Yellowish and brownish teeth are more receptive to bleaching than blue- and gray-tinged teeth. Aside from those general observations, it is difficult to know how your particular teeth will respond to bleaching. Some people have great success achieving a whiter, brighter smile after tooth bleaching. For others, the difference in tooth color after bleaching is more subtle. In general, though, most people find their teeth are one to two shades whiter after bleaching.

What is involved in bleaching?

First, the dentist makes a mold of your upper and lower teeth. The mold is used to create a soft, rubberized applicator tray similar to a tooth protector worn by football players and other athletes, but much thinner. This whole process can be completed in less than an hour. Your tray differs from the athletic tooth protector in that it will have a series of small, strategically located reservoirs to hold bleaching gel against selected teeth. The teeth selected for bleaching are generally the front teeth and any premolars and molars that can be seen when you smile broadly.

Along with the applicator tray, you will receive an adequate supply of bleaching gel—a thick, viscous material whose active ingredient is carbamide peroxide. The pleasant-tasting gels come in a variety of concentrations such as 10, 15, and 22 percent. Your dentist will determine an appropriate concentration based on your current tooth color, the likely causes of tooth discoloration, and how white you wish to go. The dentist will instruct you on how to fill the tray with enough gel to do the job but not so much that it will ooze into your mouth.

It is recommended that you wear the applicator tray at least one to two hours a night, or you may sleep with the gel-filled tray in your mouth. Be sure to brush your teeth right before inserting the tray. Brushing removes plaque, making more of your teeth's surface area accessible to the bleaching gel. You'll also want to rinse and brush well after removing the tray to avoid swallowing the gel or letting it sit on your gums.

Most people attain optimal bleaching after two weeks of nightly use.

How much does tooth bleaching cost?

Most dentists charge anywhere from $200 to $400 for a take-home tooth-bleaching system. Remember that you are paying for the dentist's time, expertise, and materials—not for a specific result.

What is "power bleaching"?

Power bleaching is a more intensive, and expensive, version of tooth bleaching that can be completed in a single office visit. It is appropriate for people who don't wish to wear the tray night after night, or who want to get a running start on their home-bleaching routine.

The gel used for power bleaching is about 35 percent hydrogen peroxide and is more caustic than the bleach formulated for home use. Before applying the bleach, the dentist will position a "dental dam" in your mouth. A dental dam is a thin, rubber sheet designed to isolate the teeth to be bleached and protect your lips and gums from the bleaching agent. The bleach is then carefully applied to the teeth and left on for seven to nine minutes. Like the home-bleaching system, power bleaching usually renders the teeth one to two shades whiter.

How much does power bleaching cost?

Because of the additional time and labor involved, dentists charge in the neighborhood of $200 to $800 per session for power bleaching.

Are there any possible adverse side effects to either power bleaching or home bleaching?

No matter how hard a dentist works to isolate the teeth for power bleaching, some of the bleach can still come into contact with the gums, turning them white. This also may cause some itchiness. Fortunately, gums are a very resilient tissue; the whiteness and itchiness usually disappear within a couple of hours.

Some people using the home-bleaching system have complained about a burning sensation in their gums. If this happens to you, using a fluoride rinse for a couple of days should alleviate the problem.

Don't worry if you inadvertently swallow some of the bleaching gel. Hydrogen peroxide has been used for many years as a treatment for canker sores, and there have been no reports of gastrointestinal distress when small amounts are ingested. Some dentists have asserted that hydrogen peroxide gel can dry out a tooth, but there is no proof that this happens.

Are the results of tooth-bleaching permanent?

If you take very good care of your teeth, the bleaching effect can last for many years. Many dentists have found that a monthly touchup with the home-bleaching kit can help sustain the whiteness. However, there is a decent chance that the discoloration will return if you continue to smoke or drink excessive amounts of coffee or tea.

What kinds of people typically seek tooth bleaching?

Bleaching is sought by a cross section of people ranging in age from their early twenties to sixties and seventies.

What if my teeth are still discolored after bleaching?

If you are still dissatisfied with the results, you can try a stronger bleach or more drastic measures, such as bonding or porcelain veneers.

What is bonding?

Bonding is a multipurpose cosmetic procedure that can whiten, close spaces, and accomplish some minor recontouring of the teeth. The technique uses a "composite"— a type of resin, or glue, infused with microscopic quartz chips—which is applied to the front of selected teeth like putty. Once on the teeth, the composite is cured (hardened) by exposure to a halogen incandescent light. It can then be shaped and polished. The whole process is completed in a single office visit that can last thirty minutes to an hour, depending on how many teeth are bonded. The composite used for bonding is the same material used to fill cavities aesthetically.

Bonding becomes a more effective, natural-looking tooth whitener if you bleach your teeth first. The whiter your teeth are to begin with, the less composite you'll need to finish the job. Badly stained teeth need a thicker coat of composite material, which makes the teeth more opaque. As translucency is lost, the teeth begin to look less vital and more fake, almost like Chiclets.

Are bonded teeth more vulnerable to stains than natural teeth?

Yes. The surface of bonded teeth can never be made as smooth as enamel or porcelain. Tiny irregularities in the bonding material are vulnerable to stains. To keep your bonded teeth as white as possible for as long as possible, avoid tobacco products, tea, and coffee and be sure to brush and floss your teeth after every meal. You should also have your teeth professionally cleaned and polished every six months. Having regular dental checkups can detect any gaps that may form between the composite and your natural tooth—gaps that can invite tooth decay.

Will my teeth feel any different after bonding?

Yes, especially if the bonding changes the teeth's dimensions in any way. The teeth's texture may also change. No matter how thoroughly your dentist polishes the hardened composite material, it may not feel quite as smooth as your natural teeth. Within a few weeks, you will grow accustomed to the new feel of your bonded teeth and won't notice any difference.

How much does bonding cost?

Most dentists charge between $200 and $250 per tooth. The number of teeth bonded usually varies from two to ten, depending on the patient's aesthetic demands.

How long does bonding last?

Bonding can last eight to ten years or longer, depending on how much stress the bonded teeth are subjected to.

How does bonding compare with porcelain veneers?

Porcelain veneers—custom designed pieces of thin porcelain that are attached to the front of teeth—have several advantages over bonding. First and foremost, veneers provide a smoother, more natural-looking result. Virtually impervious to stain, veneers are stronger and less likely to chip or break than bonded teeth. Porcelain veneers should last longer than bonding, if you take care of them. From the dentist's perspective, veneers provide greater control and flexibility when it comes to reshaping the teeth; in addition to closing spaces and giving teeth a better contour, porcelain veneers can make the teeth longer—something bonding cannot do as predictably or reliably.

All these advantages come at a cost: At $500 to $700 per tooth, porcelain veneers are about three times more expensive than bonding. Veneers are more costly because the process requires two visits to the dentist and involves a lab fee.

For Robert, a sixty-year-old stockbroker, a new, improved smile was well worth the expense. "They're fabulous," he says of his veneers. "My wife is jealous."

Robert initially got veneers on his two upper front teeth because they were crooked. But that created a contrast between his dazzling white front teeth and the rest of his mouth. Three months later, Robert was back in the prosthodontist's chair having ten more teeth done.

"It took a couple of days to get used to them," he said. "But now, I don't feel any difference."

How are porcelain veneers applied?

Tooth preparation followed by the creation and application of porcelain veneers require two office visits. During the first visit, the dentist makes two impressions of your teeth that will be used to create molds. The molds are necessary to make temporary and permanent veneers. After the first impression is made, your teeth are numbed with injections of local anesthetic. The dentist then grinds away approximately three-quarters of a millimeter of the enamel layer from the front of each tooth that is to receive a veneer. The grinding covers the whole visible portion of the tooth down to a point just below the gum line. After the grinding, the second impression is made. Using both molds, the dentist fashions temporary plastic veneers that will cover the teeth for about a week—the time it takes for a dental lab to manufacture permanent porcelain veneers. The temporary veneers, or "temps," are cemented to the tooth and should not affect your teeth's function. Any pain or discomfort in your gums after the first visit can usually be controlled with acetaminophen.

When the permanent veneers are ready, you return to the office. The temporary veneers are removed, and the porcelain veneers are attached to the teeth using a material similar to the composite used for tooth bonding. The veneers are then adjusted and polished.

Unless the shape or contour of your veneers is to be altered, both the temporary and permanent veneers must be precisely measured to replace the exact amount of enamel that was removed—about three-quarters of a millimeter. At the very least, the shape of veneer that touches the gums must match the shape and contour of the enamel it is replacing. This maintains the integrity of the region where gum and tooth material meet. If the spatial relationship between the tooth shape and surrounding gum is changed, gum disease can result.

Robert, the stockbroker, wishes he had demanded higher quality temporary veneers when he had his first two teeth done. "They loosened up, and I had to make an extra trip to the office to have them cemented in again," he recalls. "That was the only inconvenience of the whole procedure."

What is microabrasion?

Microabrasion is a way of removing tooth stains that are confined to the outer surface of the tooth enamel and cannot be corrected through bleaching. The dentist first isolates the stained tooth or teeth with a dental dam. Using a hand-held, low-speed polishing tool equipped with a rubber cup to prevent splashing, the dentist polishes the stains with a material made of pumice mixed with hydrochloric acid. Enamel is removed in tiny increments until the stain is gone. Microabrasion generally takes five to ten minutes per tooth. If the stain is deeper than anticipated, the dentist may need to switch to bonding or a veneer.

How much does it cost?

Microabrasion costs about $50 to $100 per tooth.

What is cosmetic contouring?

Cosmetic contouring is basically sculpting a tooth to give it a more aesthetically pleasing shape. You might use cosmetic contouring to take a point off a canine tooth, round off a corner of a central incisor to give it a softer shape, or make your teeth blend in better with the curvature of your lips when you smile.

Cosmetic contouring is done with a slowly rotating grinding stone as you watch the action in a mirror. The dentist takes away tooth a tiny bit at a time until you are satisfied. The goal is to make your teeth look great without being obvious that you had some help from a grinding stone.

Cosmetic contouring is a one-visit procedure. The procedure can take anywhere from a few minutes to an hour, depending on how many teeth are being contoured. No anesthesia is needed.

What does cosmetic contouring cost?

Most dentists charge $50 to $100 per tooth, depending on how much time the procedure requires.

What if my teeth look okay but my gums are red and swollen?

Proper tooth-brushing technique, a Waterpik, and special mouthwashing can prevent most gingival (gum) problems. In severe cases where the gums have shrunken, exposing roots of the teeth, periodontists use techniques to move gum tissue to cover the defects.

When I smile, I have too much gum showing. Can anything be done?

Here, the periodontist can work in concert with a plastic surgeon to reduce excess gum tissue and, perhaps, lower the upper lip. In people with tooth loss, proper dentures can be fitted to plump out the cheek and lips and even push out a recessed upper lip.

What other cosmetic dental techniques are available?

Orthodontia is used to straighten out crooked teeth and improve the bite and appearance. The importance of replacing missing teeth with removable or permanent dentures cannot be overemphasized.

ETCETERA

Spider Veins, Moles, and Scars

What is a spider vein?

A spider vein is actually a tiny blood vessel called a capillary that is visible through the skin. The red, weblike structures you see are not the actual clear-walled capillaries, but the blood flowing through them. Spider veins occur primarily on the legs and thighs but can occur on the face, as well. Although considered unattractive, spider veins are completely harmless.

Spider veins should not be confused with larger, bluish varicose veins, whose treatment is generally considered outside the realm of cosmetic surgery. If you want to get rid of varicose veins, the entire venous system of your legs and thighs should first be evaluated by a vascular surgeon to determine whether treatment is indicated.

What causes spider veins?

A variety of factors could be to blame. On the lower extremities, spider veins are often caused by the effects of gravity. If you stand on your feet for long periods of time, you are particularly vulnerable. Hormones—especially those associated with pregnancy—also play a role, as do your genes.

Some people have a genetic tendency for spider veins on the face. People who smoke, drink alcohol regularly, or eat an abundance of spicy foods have a higher likelihood of developing facial spider veins. In some cases, facial spider veins mark the onset of a chronic skin disease called acne rosacea, which later develops into abnormal redness of the nose and cheeks, along with pimples and thickened skin.

Once a spider vein appears, it is there to stay unless it is treated.

How are spider veins removed from the legs?

The proven method of removing spider veins from the lower legs and thighs is by injecting them with a very strong saltwater solution (saline), or one of a variety of other chemicals, the most common being sodium morrhuate. All the chemicals yield similar results, although the advantage of saline is that there is no potential for an allergic reaction.

Using strong magnification and intense light trained on the affected area, the doctor begins the procedure by applying alcohol to the skin. Alcohol makes the spider veins more visible even as it sterilizes. Using an extraordinarily thin, handmade needle, the doctor (a dermatologist, plastic surgeon, or vascular surgeon) injects a tiny droplet of fluid into the spider vein. Usually, one-tenth of a milliliter is all that is needed per capillary. The goal is to flush out the blood and damage the inner lining of the vessel. Almost immediately after injection, the capillary walls swell. Hopefully, the inner wall of the capillary will adhere to the opposing inner wall as it heals. To help the healing process along, the doctor may apply pressure by taping cotton balls over the injection site. Wearing a special compressive stocking for forty-eight hours after treatment further increases the chance that the treated capillaries will remain closed. When this happens, the spider vein disappears for good.

Does the procedure hurt?

You will feel a tiny sting as the needle enters your skin followed by a brief burning sensation as the solution is injected. No anesthetic is needed because the needles are so thin—thin enough to fit inside the capillary. Injecting a local anesthetic would be more painful than the treatment.

How long does the treatment take?

Because most people have multiple spider veins, treatment is normally done in a series of sessions lasting about forty-five minutes. Injecting an individual spider vein can take as little as ten seconds, depending on the doctor's skill. Capillaries are interconnected, like the branches of a tree. If the doctor can inject the base of a branch, it is possible to destroy up to ten spider veins with a single injection. Experienced physicians can treat dozens, if not hundreds, of spider veins per session.

Are the results immediate?

Some capillaries will be instantly obliterated upon injection, while others may stay visible for four weeks before disappearing. In the latter cases, capillary blood gets trapped between the collapsed entrance and exit of the vessel but is digested by the body over the next month. Conversely, some spider veins that disappear during the treatment session may reappear several weeks later. This occasionally happens because the body is very adept at keeping capillaries open and reopening ones that have collapsed.

The bottom line of all this uncertainty is to wait at least a month before deciding whether to retreat spider veins.

What are the risks of treatment?

There could be a scar should the chemical leak out of the capillary and damage the skin. Fortunately, this does not happen often. More common is temporary blistering of the treatment area. Some patients develop a brownish stain on the skin, which is caused by blood leaking out of the capillary. In most cases, the stain fades in six months, although some stains are permanent. Infection as a result of injection therapy is extremely rare.

Patients must realize that treating today's spider veins in no way affects their risk of developing new spider veins in the future. The process of spider-vein formation is ongoing since the same forces that cause them—gravity, genetics, and lifestyle—are still at work.

How much does it cost to remove spider veins from legs?

Doctors' fees vary widely, with some charging more than $400 for a forty-five-minute treatment session. A pair of good surgical stockings can cost you more than $100 if they are thigh-high.

How are spider veins removed from the face?

There are two accepted methods of treatment: electrocoagulation and laser. For either technique, your face first will be numbed with EMLA cream, a topical anesthetic.

In electrocoagulation, the doctor uses a needle like the ones used for electrolysis. The needle is placed through the skin into the capillary, and a low-voltage electrical current is passed through the needle, destroying the capillary.

The more modern approach employs one of a number of new lasers, such as the "pulse dye laser" or "copper vapor laser," both of which heat the blood in the spider vein and damage the capillary's inner wall. The reason laser and electrocoagulation don't work on the lower extremities is probably because of the effects of gravity, which are not present on the face.

A new treatment, which was introduced in early 1996 with great fanfare, is similar to a laser but is not a true laser because it emits high-intensity light of multiple wavelengths instead of a single wavelength. Although this new $80,000 piece of medical equipment has received much publicity, many plastic surgeons have questioned its effectiveness, citing results that show minimal improvement of leg spider veins. When patients undergo treatment, they want all their spider veins gone, not just some of them.

Will a scar be left behind?

Neither laser treatment nor electrocoagulation should leave behind a scar. There may be tiny porelike depressions created from electrocoagulation, similar to the depressions created from electrolysis and dark spots from prolonged bruising.

Are there other possible complications of electrocoagulation or laser treatment?

In men, there is a chance of hair loss in the vicinity of the treated facial spider vein, although this is less likely to occur with the laser method. Infection would be very unlikely. Scarring, reoccurrence, or incomplete removal of the spider vein are other risks.

What do these treatments cost?

Electrocoagulation, which is usually done in the doctor's office, varies in cost depending on the number of spider veins treated. All facial spider veins often can be treated in one session costing between $200 and $500.

Laser treatment can cost up to four times as much: generally $700 or $800 per treatment session. In most cases, laser therapy is done in a hospital on an outpatient basis. The lasers used to treat spider veins carry a price tag of about $150,000—an investment that few medical practitioners can justify.

Will the skin where a facial spider vein was removed look any different from surrounding skin?

It should not.

Are there any steps I can take to reduce my future risk for spider veins?

Don't drink. Don't smoke. And don't get pregnant. Even if you observe all these measures, there is still a very good chance that more spider veins will appear within a year or two.

Are there any medical reasons for getting rid of spider veins?

No. Treatment is done for purely aesthetic reasons.

Are there any therapeutic reasons for removing a mole?

Yes. Certain types of moles can become malignant melanomas, a potentially deadly form of skin cancer. Also, a melanoma can be mistaken for a mole, which puts a person's life at risk if the lesion is not removed in time.

For these reasons, as well as for cosmetic reasons, many moles should be removed. The question is, which mole? In general, a mole should be surgically removed if

1. it is greater than one-quarter inch in diameter;
2. it has an irregular border;
3. it contains more than one color, such as light brown and dark brown, or dark brown and black;
4. it bleeds, itches, or undergoes other changes;
5. the mole is blue in color; or
6. you have had the mole since birth.

Statistically, a mole you are born with has a 4 to 9 percent chance of becoming malignant during your lifetime. There is no peak year for this to happen; the malignancy can develop during your first year of life or your seventieth. It is therefore important to have these moles removed as soon as is feasible.

When a dermatologist identifies a suspicious mole, it is

labeled "atypical." Atypical moles should be watched closely by the patient and carefully examined by a dermatologist every six months. A mole has a much higher likelihood of becoming a melanoma if the disease runs in your family or you have had a malignant melanoma elsewhere on your body.

If every mole is a potential melanoma, why not have them all removed?

This would be impractical, not to mention cost-prohibitive. Virtually everyone has twenty to thirty moles; there aren't enough doctors in the country to remove them all. So moles are removed only if they look suspicious, have changed, or are cosmetically undesirable by the patient.

What exactly is a mole?

A mole, technically known as a "nevus," is darkly colored, raised, benign (nonmalignant) tumor of the pigment-producing cells of skin, or melanocytes. Moles are different from café au lait spots, which are lightly pigmented and flat. If there is a question, a biopsy can be performed on a tiny piece of the lesion to determine its true nature.

Which doctors routinely remove moles?

Dermatologists and plastic surgeons probably do the vast majority of mole removal in this country. Some family practitioners also remove moles. If your mole is situated on a cosmetically sensitive area, such as your face or breasts, you would probably be referred to a plastic surgeon to have it removed.

How are moles removed?

Moles should not be shaved, frozen, or lasered off the skin. The only proper way to remove a mole is to "excise" it—cut it off. If a mole is removed by any other means, it can grow back and look like a cancer.

After sterilizing the area and injecting a local anesthetic, the doctor makes an incision, usually elliptical, around the mole. Plastic surgeons, in particular, try to place the incision along a natural wrinkle line or border of an anatomical structure such as the areola junction, base of the nose, or in front of the ear. This makes the scar less noticeable. After the mole is removed, the skin surrounding the wound is undermined (lifted) one-quarter inch to one inch to allow the skin to stretch. The incision is then closed with at least two layers of sutures: dissolving sutures in the dermis and fine, removable stitches on the surface of the skin. The surface sutures are not tied too tightly and are removed by seven days in order to minimize cross marks and suture points in the skin.

Does the mole removal procedure hurt?
There may be some degree of discomfort, depending on the skills of the surgeon and the sensitivity of the area being operated on. There is a small amount of pain associated with the injection of local anesthetic.

How long does it take?
Anywhere from ten minutes to an hour, depending on the size, depth, and location of the mole.

Are moles routinely examined for malignant cells, even if they are not suspicious?
Yes, this is required by law in most states. It would be considered malpractice not to have an excised mole evaluated under a microscope by a pathologist.

How bad will my scar be?
It depends on where your mole was located. Some parts of the body, such as the upper middle chest, are notoriously bad for scars. If you have a mole removed from your chest, there will be a 20 percent chance of having an unattractive scar. That compares with a 2 percent chance of a bad scar

if the mole was removed from your eyelid. Other areas of the face also usually heal with minimal scarring.

What are the possible complications of mole removal?

Most procedures are done without incident, but there is a small risk of infection or bleeding any time the skin is opened. There is also a tiny risk of having an adverse reaction to the local anesthetic. If the mole is not removed properly, there is a risk of it growing back. Bad scarring is another potential problem.

How much does mole removal cost?

Again, doctors' fees vary, with facial moles being generally more expensive to remove than moles on other areas. A family doctor may charge around $200 for mole removal. Most plastic surgeons will not do the procedure for less than $500. Dermatologists generally charge somewhere in between. Because any mole has the potential of becoming malignant, it is not unusual for medical insurance to cover the procedure in full or in part.

How are café au lait spots removed?

Like freckles or blotchy brown spots, café au lait spots can be safely removed by laser (see Chapter Seven), chemical peel (see Chapter Six), dermabrasion (see Chapter Six), skin bleaching (see Chapter Six), or freezing with liquid nitrogen.

Can unsightly scars stemming from surgery or accidents be made less noticeable?

Yes, in certain cases, with a procedure known as "scar revision." Contrary to popular belief, plastic surgeons cannot remove or erase scars completely. Scar revision can, however, make unsightly or unattractive scars less unattractive.

What happens during a scar revision procedure?

The basic strategy is to excise the unsightly scar, lift up the skin edges to reduce tension, and close the wound with two layers of stitches, just as a plastic surgeon would close the wound after a mole removal. Whenever possible, the new incision is realigned to fall into a wrinkle line or made to fall in a natural boundary between anatomic structures. A scar may be lengthened if it is tethering adjacent structures, or it may be broken up into a series of shorter lines.

If the scar is raised, the surgeon can flatten it with dermabrasion (see Chapter Six) or a laser (see Chapter Seven). The same CO_2 laser used for laser peels can also shrink scars, including shallow acne scars, although recent reports suggest that effect may be temporary. Large, broad areas of scar can be replaced with skin grafts, flaps of adjacent tissue, skin expanded with the aid of special balloons, or tissue transferred from remote locations with the aid of microsurgery.

What exactly is scar tissue, and how does it differ from normal skin?

Scar tissue is to the body what spackle is to plaster walls. Making scar tissue is the body's reparative response to injury. Like skin, scar tissue is comprised primarily of collagen, but it is less organized. Because of that, scar tissue can never be as strong as normal skin or as aesthetically pleasing, but it is certainly better than nothing.

Why does the appearance of scars change?

Scars go through a "maturation" process that normally takes an entire year. During the first three months, the body puts lots and lots of scar tissue into a wound to increase the scar's strength. The scar becomes hard, red, and raised. After the first three months, the body ceases making scar tissue and starts to "remodel" the scar. The scar gradually softens and turns from red to pink and ultimately to flesh toned, although people with darkly pigmented skin often produce scars that are darker than surrounding skin. At the same time, the raised portion of the scar settles down.

There are always exceptions to the normal course of events. Some people take longer for scar maturation, and others take less time; some people develop scars that almost look like normal skin. Others end up with unattractive scars. Also, how you scar on one part of the body does not necessarily predict how you will scar on another part.

What are the risks of scar revision?

There is a small risk of infection and minor bleeding. There is also a risk that your scar will look worse than it did to begin with.

How much does the procedure cost?

The range of costs varies as much as the appearance of scars. The least expensive procedure might be a spot dermabrasion of a single scar, which runs several hundred dollars. Very complicated reconstructive surgery to remove significant scars can exceed $10,000.

What kind of scars respond best to scar revision?

Any unattractive scar would benefit from scar revision if it stems from a wound that was not treated or was not sewn up by a board-certified plastic surgeon or other doctor familiar with meticulous techniques. Conversely, scar-revision techniques are probably useless if your scar resulted from work by a board-certified plastic surgeon. If you experienced a bad result from one plastic surgeon, it is unlikely that another plastic surgeon can make it any better. In such cases, the bad result probably stems from your genetic destiny as opposed to poor surgical technique.

There are a couple of exceptions. When scars result from surgical incisions that were sewn together under a lot of tension, it is often possible to make improvements once the scar has fully matured and the skin has had time to stretch.

For example, large scars resulting from breast reductions and tummy tucks can be cut away and the skin sewn closed again under far less tension than before. Such a revision often results in much smaller scars.

What is the success rate of scar revision?

Success rates vary too widely from patient to patient and scar to scar to make any meaningful generalizations. Any scar revision has one of three possible results: It makes the scar look better, it leaves it unchanged, or it makes it worse. Ask your surgeon to estimate the likelihood of each of these possible outcomes. Only then can you make an informed decision on whether to have the procedure done.

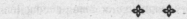

GLOSSARY

abdominoplasty: see *tummy tuck*.

aesthetic surgery: type of plastic surgery performed solely to improve appearance.

alpha-hydroxy acid: mild acid derived from certain fruits and other foods that removes surface cells when applied to skin.

ambulatory surgical facility: operating room outside of a hospital setting where patients can spend up to twenty-three hours.

anesthesiologist: medical doctor specializing in the administration of medications that put patients to sleep during surgery and monitoring patients during surgery.

aneurysm: bulge that forms in a weakened section of an artery.

areola: pigmented region around the nipple.

arrhythmia: irregular heart rhythm.

autologous fat grafts: wrinkle-filler made from a patient's own fat taken from another body site.

betadine: liquid disinfectant used to sterilize the skin prior to surgery.

blepharoplasty: see *eyelid-lift*.

body contouring: umbrella term for a variety of procedures that reshape the body by removing or manipulating fat, skin, and muscle.

bonding: application of a white composite material to teeth to improve their color, shape, or alignment.

botulinum toxin: poison derived from bacteria that causes botulism; injected to temporarily paralyze overactive muscles.

bovine collagen: fibrous protein derived from cow hide that is used to fill lines and wrinkles.

breast augmentation: surgery to enlarge the breasts by inserting implants.

breast-lift: surgical procedure that removes excess skin, elevates nipples, and tightens breast tissue to restore a normal contour to sagging breasts; also known as mastopexy.

brow-lift: see *forehead-lift*.

buttock-lift: surgical procedure to remove excess skin and fat from the buttock region and redrape remaining skin to make sagging buttocks tighter.

cannula: blunt-ended hollow tube used to break up and vacuum fat during liposuction.

canthopexy: surgery to shorten the lower eyelids' length horizontally.

capsular contracture: condition in which a wall of scar tissue that normally grows around breast implants squeezes them, making the breasts hard, and in some cases, distorting their appearance.

cellulite: visible manifestation of fibrous bands that tether skin to underlying muscle; more prevalent in aged, sagging skin.

chemabrasion: a skin-removal method that combines a chemical peel with dermabrasion.

chemical peel: applying chemicals to the face to remove superficial fine lines, multiple wrinkles, and irregular pigmentation; also known as chemosurgery.

chemosurgery: see *chemical peel*.

chin augmentation: see *mentoplasty*.

collagen: strong fibrous protein that holds all the body's tissues together.

columella: skin bridge separating the nostrils.

composite face-lift: face-lifting technique in which the skin and fibrous/fatty layer are lifted as one unit.

contour deformity: defect in the skin, such as acne scars or wrinkles.

corrugator muscles: group of muscles in the forehead that, when contracted, produce vertical "frown" lines between the eyebrows.

cosmetic contouring: reshaping the teeth with a slowly rotating grinding stone.

cosmetic dentistry: a range of dental procedures that enhance the teeth's appearance without necessarily improving their function.

cosmetic surgery: see *aesthetic surgery*.

crow's feet: a series of horizontal lines at the outer corners of the eyes that usually appear only when a person smiles; also known as "laugh lines."

cyst: a noncancerous lump that can form in the skin or any other bodily organ or tissue.

dental dam: a thin rubber sheet used to protect lips and gums from tooth-bleaching chemicals.

dentin: a resilient material that constitutes the teeth's inner core.

dermabrasion: the mechanical removal of the outer layers of skin using a dermabrader, a hand-held tool with a rapidly rotating sander or wire brush.

dermatologist: a medical doctor who specializes in diseases of the skin.

dermis: the innermost layers of skin.

deviated septum: see *septum*.

dynamic wrinkles: lines or creases in the skin that are only visible when the face is animated.

ectropion: "basset-hound" appearance in which the lower eyelids are pulled down as a result of an eyelid-lift, laser peel, aging, or scarring.

elastin: microscopic fibers in the skin that control the skin's elasticity.

electrocoagulation: controlling bleeding during surgery by heat-sealing blood vessels with a high-frequency electrical current.

endoscope: tube-shaped probe fitted with a miniature video camera and tiny fiber-optic light source.

endoscopy: surgical technique that allows the surgeon to operate remotely through small incisions with the aid of a camera.

epidermis: outermost layers of skin.

epidural anesthesia: spinal block that numbs the lower half of the body.

epinephrine: adrenaline.

excise: to surgically cut away tissue from the body.

exercise stress test: diagnostic procedure that measures the heart's activity during exercise and can detect heart disease.

exfoliate: to remove the outermost layer of skin cells.

eyelid-lift: surgery to tighten sagging, wrinkled, or hooded eyelids; also known as blepharoplasty.

face-lift: operation that removes excess skin and tightens the lower half of the face.

Fibrel: wrinkle-filling substance derived from pig collagen.

Flexzan: a sophisticated biomembrane that retains moisture, decreases pain, and hastens healing of surgical wounds.

forehead-lift: a facial rejuvenation procedure that smooths forehead furrows, lifts sagging eyebrows, and minimizes frown lines between the eyebrows.

general anesthesia: a state of drug-induced unconsciousness designed to prevent pain and discomfort during surgery.

glycolic acid: the most popular of the alpha-hydroxy acids. An ingredient in many skin-care products, glycolic acid is also used for ultralight chemical peels, also known as "lunch-time peels," to rejuvenate facial skin.

graft: living tissue that is transplanted from one part of the body to another, from one person to another person, or from an animal to a human.

gynecomastia: an often transient condition in which one or both male breasts swell, usually due to a hormonal imbalance.

hematoma: localized bleeding or blood clot under the skin.

herpes: one of various conditions that produces small, often painful skin blisters.

high lateral tension abdominoplasty: tummy tuck done through an incision across the lower belly angling sharply upward at the sides.

hydroquinones: a class of chemicals used in skin bleaches.

injectable fillers: material that is implanted or injected beneath the skin's surface to plump up lines, wrinkles, creases, and depressions, or to make the lips fuller.

intraoral photography: a system of taking detailed pictures of the teeth.

jowls: loose skin and excess fat that hang off the sides of the lower jaw.

laser peel: a facial rejuvenation technique that uses a pulsed carbon dioxide laser to vaporize outer skin layers and tighten the underlying collagen.

lidocaine: the most commonly used local anesthetic.

light chemical peel: see *trichloracetic acid.*

lip augmentation: an autologous fat transplant or implant into the lips to make them more plump.

liposuction: a procedure that removes excess fat by suctioning it out of the body; also known as "lipectomy," "liposculpture," and "lipoplasty."

liquid silicone: an injectable filling agent that was used in the past but is now illegal due to serious safety concerns.

local anesthesia: medicinally induced numbness of a limited area of the body to prevent pain and discomfort during surgery or other medical procedures.

malar bones: cheekbones.

mammography: a low-dose x-ray of the breasts designed to detect breast cancer.

mastectomy: surgery to remove all the breast tissue.

mastopexy: see *breast-lift*.

melanin: a pigment in the skin that protects the body from ultraviolet light.

melanocyte: a melanin-producing skin cell.

melanoma: a potentially fatal form of skin cancer.

mentoplasty: surgery to implant a piece of solid silicone to enlarge a chin that is too small; also known as chin augmentation.

microabrasion: removal of superficial stains from tooth enamel using a low-speed polishing tool.

micropigmentation: cosmetic tattooing, such as permanent eyeliner.

milia: tiny whiteheads on the skin caused by clogged pores.

mole: a noncancerous tumor of the pigment-producing cells of skin; also known as a nevus.

nasolabial folds: deep vertical creases that run between the nostrils and the corners of the mouth.

neurologist: a medical doctor specializing in diseases of the brain and nervous system.

nevus: see *mole*.

nonsteroidal anti-inflammatory drugs: a class of drugs including ibuprofen, diflunisal, fenoprofen, and meclofenamate, which kills pain and reduces inflammation.

ophthalmologist: a medical doctor who specializes in diseases of the eye.

orbital septum: a membrane within the eye socket that holds in place a series of protective fat pads.

orthopedist: a medical doctor who specializes in disorders of the bones, joints, ligaments, and tendons.

otolaryngologist: a surgeon who specializes in structures of the head and neck.

otoplasty: a surgical procedure to tack protruding ears back into a normal position.

outpatient surgery: any operation that allows the patient to go home in twenty-three hours or less; also known as "day surgery" and "ambulatory surgery."

parrot beak: a deformity in which abnormal fullness forms above the tip of the nose; also known as "polly beak."

pectoralis muscle: a chest muscle responsible for moving the arm forward and inward.

periodontist: a dentist who specializes in gum disease.

perioral: the area around the mouth.

periosteum: a thin but strong layer of tissue that covers the bones.

phenol peel: a deep chemical skin peel using carbolic acid.

photoaging: accelerated skin aging that results from the cumulative effects of unprotected exposure to the sun's ultraviolet radiation.

plastic surgeon: a medical doctor who specializes in surgical procedures that change a person's appearance or function.

plastic surgery: a type of surgery that molds the human body into a new form.

platysmaplasty: a surgical repair of the neck muscles that involves sewing the two ends of the muscles together, creating one continuous muscle instead of a pair of prominent cords ("turkey-gobbler neck").

porcelain veneers: custom-made porcelain shells that are attached to the front of teeth to make the smile whiter and more uniform.

power bleaching: a strong tooth-whitening technique that combines home and office bleaching applications.

prosthodontist: a dentist who specializes in tooth-replacement procedures.

reconstructive surgery: a type of plastic surgery that is performed to improve or restore function and appearance in deformed, injured, or diseased tissues.

rectus muscles: the straight, vertically oriented abdominal muscles.

reduction mammoplasty: surgery to reduce oversized

breasts so they are more proportional to the rest of the body; also known as breast-reduction surgery.

restrictive garment: a very tight girdle that is worn after certain kinds of surgery to reduce swelling and bruising.

rhinoplasty: a type of cosmetic surgery that reshapes the nose.

rhytidectomy: face-lift.

saline breast implant: silicone-rubber bag filled with salt-water used to enlarge the breasts; currently the only legal breast implant in the United States.

scleroderma: a rare autoimmune disease that can attack the skin and internal organs. Symptoms include ultrasensitivity to cold and hardening of the tissues.

scrub nurse: an operating room nurse who is cleansed and dressed appropriately to work within a sterile operating field.

septal reconstruction: a surgical procedure to correct a deviated septum severe enough to cause breathing problems.

septum: the wall made of cartilage that separates the nostril chambers; when it is off the midline, it is called a "deviated septum."

shingles: a skin infection that affects the nerves that supply specific areas of the skin. Also known as herpes zoster, shingles stems from the same virus that causes chickenpox.

skin necrosis: a postsurgical complication in which skin cells die because they were robbed of their blood supply.

skin resurfacing: any procedure that removes old skin to allow new, younger-looking skin to grow back in its place.

sliding genioplasty: surgical correction of a severely undersized chin by cutting the chin bone and moving it forward, backward, up, or down with metal plates and titanium screws.

SPF (sun-protection factor): a number that indicates the strength of a sunscreen or sunblock; the higher a product's number, the more protection it provides from the sun's harmful ultraviolet rays.

static wrinkles: lines or creases in the skin that are visible when the facial muscles are relaxed.

submalar implants: pieces of solid silicone placed just under the cheekbones to plump up hollow cheeks.

subperiosteal face-lift: a face-lifting technique that undermines the skin and all underlying tissues clear to the level of bone.

surgical rejuvenation: cosmetic surgery that makes people look like they did when they were younger.

surgicenter: a freestanding medical facility where outpatient surgery is performed.

thigh-lift: a surgical procedure that tightens sagging skin on the inner thighs, outer thighs, or both.

tooth bleaching: a home-based system of applying a bleaching gel to teeth in order to make them whiter.

transconjunctival eyelid-lift: lower eyelid-lift done through an incision inside the lid.

trichloracetic acid: a chemical used for light face peels; also known as TCA.

tumescent liposuction: a liposuction technique in which an epinephrine-containing anesthetic solution is first injected under the skin.

tummy tuck: an operation to flatten the protruding belly by removing excess skin and fat and, if necessary, sewing the abdominal muscles together to create an ''inner girdle''; also known as abdominoplasty.

ultralight chemical peel: see *glycolic acid*.

ultrapulsed laser: a specialized laser that delivers high-energy light in tiny bursts.

ultrasound-assisted liposuction (UAL): a fat-suctioning technique in which ultrasonic waves are used to emulsify fat before it is vacuumed away.

undermine: lifting one layer of tissue from an underlying layer of tissue or bone.

vasoconstrictor: any drug whose main effect or side effect narrows blood vessels.

Zovirax: an antiviral drug used in the treatment and prevention of herpes breakouts.

APPENDIX A

Boards That Are Recognized By the American Board of Medical Specialties

The American Board of Allergy and Immunology, Inc.
The American Board of Anesthesiology, Inc.
The American Board of Colon and Rectal Surgery, Inc.
The American Board of Dermatology, Inc.
The American Board of Emergency Medicine, Inc.
The American Board of Family Practice, Inc.
The American Board of Internal Medicine, Inc.
The American Board of Medical Genetics, Inc.
The American Board of Neurological Surgery, Inc.
The American Board of Nuclear Medicine, Inc.
The American Board of Obstetrics and Gynecology, Inc.
The American Board of Ophthalmology, Inc.
The American Board of Orthopaedic Surgery, Inc.
The American Board of Otolaryngology, Inc.
The American Board of Pathology, Inc.
The American Board of Pediatrics, Inc.
The American Board of Physical Medicine and
   Rehabilitation, Inc.

The American Board of Plastic Surgery, Inc.
The American Board of Preventive Medicine, Inc.
The American Board of Psychiatry and Neurology, Inc.
The American Board of Radiology, Inc.
The American Board of Surgery, Inc.
The American Board of Thoracic Surgery, Inc.
The American Board of Urology, Inc.

APPENDIX B

Consultation Comparison Checklist

Date of Consultation: _____
Name of Surgeon: _____
My Complaints: _____
_____
_____
_____
_____

Procedure(s) Surgeon Suggested: _____
_____
_____
_____

FEES

Surgeon: _____
Operating Facility: _____
Anesthesia: _____
Other (implants, etc.): _____

SURGEON INFORMATION

Surgical Training: _____

Plastic Surgery Training: _____

Board Certified: Yes/No _____

Which Board: _____

Recommended by (doctor, friend, etc.): _____

OPERATING FACILITY

❑ Hospital (which one): _____

❑ Surgicenter (which one): _____

❑ Office

If office operating room, accredited by:

❑ AAAASF

❑ AAAHC

❑ Other: _____

Medicare Certified: Yes/No

ANESTHESIA BY

❑ Anesthesiologist (M.D.)

❑ Nurse Anesthetist (R.N.)

❑ Other _____

MY COMMENTS ABOUT THE SURGEON (Personality, rapport, etc.): _____

_____

_____

Robin Karol Levinson is an author, editor, writing instructor, and award-winning journalist specializing in health, science, and fitness. Her other books include *Get Your Rear In Gear* (HarperCollins), *A Woman Doctor's Guide to Osteoporosis*, and *A Woman Doctor's Guide to Infertility* (Hyperion). She lives in New Jersey with her husband, daughter, and son.

Arthur William Perry, M.D., F.A.C.S., is a board-certified plastic surgeon and medical journalist who specializes primarily in aesthetic plastic surgery. He received his Doctor of Medicine with Distinction in Research from the Albany Medical College of Union University in 1981 and trained in general surgery at Harvard Medical School's Beth Israel Hospital in Boston. He trained in burn surgery at the New York Hospital/Cornell, in plastic surgery at the University of Chicago, and in aesthetic surgery in Miami. A member of the New Jersey Board of Medical Examiners, Dr. Perry holds faculty appointments at the University of Pennsylvania School of Medicine and the University of Medicine and Dentistry of New Jersey–Robert Wood Johnson Medical School. He has received numerous awards and honors for his clinical work and research and is a member of the national medical honor society, Alpha Omega Alpha. Dr. Perry maintains a private practice in the Princeton, New Jersey area where he resides with his wife and three children.